THE COMPLETE
POSTPARTUM
GUIDE

THE COMPLETE
POSTPARTUM
GUIDE

EVERYTHING YOU NEED TO
KNOW ABOUT TAKING CARE
OF YOURSELF AFTER
YOU'VE HAD A BABY

DIANE LYNCH-FRASER

1817

HARPER & ROW, PUBLISHERS, New York
Cambridge, Philadelphia, San Francisco,
London, Mexico City, São Paulo, Sydney

Grateful acknowledgment is made for permission to reprint: Excerpt from *Unfinished Business* by Maggie Scarf reprinted by permission of Doubleday & Co., Inc. Excerpt from *Lillian Bloom: A Separation* by Judith Steinbergh, copyright © 1981 by Judith Steinbergh, reprinted by permission of Wampeter Press, Green Harbor, MA 02041. Excerpt from *Twilight of Authority* by Robert Nisbet reprinted by permission of Oxford University Press. Excerpt from *Ourselves and Our Children* by The Boston Women's Health Book Collective, Inc, copyright © 1978 by The Boston Women's Health Book Collective, Inc.

FIRST EDITION

Designer: Robin Malkin

Library of Congress Cataloging in Publication Data

Lynch-Fraser, Diane.
    The complete postpartum guide.

    Bibliography: p.
    Includes index.
    1. Postnatal care. 2. Exercises for women.
3. Mothers—Psychology. 4. Mothers—Family relationships. I. Title.
RG801.L96   1983   618.6   82–48673
ISBN 0–06–015142–0

---

83 84 85 86 87 10 9 8 7 6 5 4 3 2 1

2206101

To my grandmother
Mary Gertrude Lynch
who raised three children in a time
of both economic and social stress
and who instilled in them and their
children a sense of heritage, creativity
and warmth

CONTENTS

ACKNOWLEDGMENTS

It must be obvious to the reader that, in writing a book of this kind, I did not accomplish this task alone—this book evolved due to the cooperation of many talented and devoted people. The first of these people, whom I will never be able to thank enough, is my literary agent, Susan Zeckendorf, whose friendship and belief in me both as a writer and as a person motivated me to undertake the enormousness of this project in the first place. I thank Susan for her inspiration. The second is my editor, Sallie Coolidge, who went through the pages of my original manuscript and helped me arrive at the finished product you how have before you. I thank Sallie for her patience.

I also want to acknowledge Drs. Sujana Patipandla and Robert Marc Fink for their professional advice; Lidy Consales, my reference librarian at the New York Academy of Medicine, for researching the necessary computer files for me; and Jeffrey Stelmach for typing the original manuscript, a task for which I have no proficiency. I also wish to thank my husband, Randy, and my daughter, Skye, for putting up with me through the endless months of writing.

Last, I want to thank all the unmentioned people—the secretaries and receptionists at the Harvard, Yale, and University of Michigan medical schools who assisted me in gaining access to individuals and information regarding this subject; and especially all the mothers who took the time to answer my rather lengthy questionnaire and, as a result, helped me to gain insights other than my own about the realities of the postpartum period.

Thank you all very, very much.

AUTHOR'S NOTE

The reader should remember two things when reading this book:

●This book represents a bridge between medical research and the casual advice which surrounds the subject of postpartum recovery. This is not a medical journal, nor is it a simple account of mothers' experiences. It is intended to be a comprehensive guide written expressly for postpartum mothers, based on documented research in this area. Since I wanted this book to read like a story and at the same time to provide an authoritative view of the subject, I included all of my reference notes at the end of the text so that they would not interrupt the flow of the book. A suggested bibliography and a list of women's support groups are also included, to assist you in finding additional information on this subject and related issues.

●Though I have tried conscientiously to avoid the use of sex-stereotyped language in my text, I have found that avoiding it completely can contribute to an awkward writing style. Therefore, in the instances where the traditional singular masculine pronoun "he" could indicate either a male or a female, I have retained the masculine "he" to avoid the awkward phrase "he or she." As I indicated in my last book, *Danceplay*, I am anxiously waiting for English grammarians and linguists to develop a suitable non-sexist singular pronoun.

The purpose of this book is to make you aware of the normal progress of the postpartum period and the possible problems you may encounter. Any symptoms you may have will require an expert assessment. Of course, proper diagnosis and therapy for all symptoms connected with pregnancy and the postpartum period require your doctor's careful attention to your concerns.

INTRODUCTION

Can a Child
move in
as easily
as a cat
—Judith Steinbergh

Chances are that if you have decided to purchase a book with a title like *The Complete Postpartum Guide*, then you, like more than half of new mothers, are not quite feeling like yourself. You feel sad, tired, and a bit guilty—not at all the way you expected to feel. You may wonder why I wanted to write this book or simply why I wanted to devote an entire book to the subject of postpartum recovery. Well, as one young mother told me,

> *Having a child is the most irreversible act a woman can perform. If she doesn't like it, she can't quit, divorce her child, or start over. It is probably the only kind of decision she will make over a lifetime that is quite so final and so terrifying.*

I wanted to give women specific information about postpartum recovery so they *would know* what to expect. I know that I could have benefited enormously had I had access to this information when I was a new mother.

I would like to begin by relating a little of my own experiences and observations and how I came to write this book in the first place. I was, for most of my young life, a professional dancer and teacher. I went to medical school, studied dance therapy, and became a certified psychomotor therapist—that is, a specialist who uses movement and music to communicate with severely physically, mentally, or emotionally handicapped people who are not able to communicate in the traditional sense. After several years as an independent teacher and as a practicing movement therapist, I became interested in teaching dance exercise. I met two former ballet dancers and began to teach for them in their Manhattan dance-exercise studio. I soon found myself managing their exercise studio, which began to specialize in prenatal and postpartum exercise classes. I also found myself pregnant!

During my three years as a pregnancy and postpartum exercise consultant, I came into contact with literally hundreds of pregnant women and postpartum mothers. I noticed that the emotional patterns among them were almost indistinguishable. They would arrive at the onset of their pregnancy jubilantly "blooming with anticipation." Their cheeks were flushed and their eyes glowing! They could have conquered the world with their enthusiasm. They were going to be "supermoms." They would be doting mothers, successful career women, interesting wives, and they were going to do it all without creasing their Laura Ashley dresses. I observed them, with their increasingly pear-shaped bodies, as they giggled over their clumsiness and lack of appetite control. They seemed to possess an unabashed energy. They would race through their prenatal exercises and then bound across the street to the local health-food emporium and indulge in a helping of frozen yogurt with granola. They were pampered women, and they enjoyed being pampered. After all, everyone loves a pregnant woman!

As the women due to deliver disappeared from exercise class, I and the other class members would await the outcome. Was it a boy or a girl? How much did it weigh? How was the delivery? We all waited for the joyful mother to return to post-partum exercise, babe in arms. I observed, however, that they did not return as quickly as they had promised. Some did not return at all. When they did return, they did not resemble their exuberant former selves. They were tired and pale, and they had a dismayed look pasted on their faces that seemed to say, "What has happened to me?" Yet they seemed to be afraid to ask that very question. Someone might accuse them of being unfit mothers. They wanted to be like the mothers in the Pampers and baby-powder commercials—young, beautiful, meticulous about every detail of their babies' lives. And what was the matter with their babies? They didn't look like the adorable infants in the Health Tex ads. Nobody had told them that the women doing the commercials are not postpartum mothers and that the babies in the ads look that way only for two minutes—then they spit up just as other babies do.

Even with my experience with pregnant and postpartum mothers, I was unprepared for my own baby, and deep down inside I knew it—but no one would talk to me about it. I remember that during my childbirth-preparation classes the obstetrical nurse who conducted the classes (a woman who, incidentally, had never had children) asked everyone to voice her greatest fear about childbirth. The women in my class voiced worries about the pain in labor, whether the child would be normal, if they would get to the hospital in time, and so on. When my turn came, I asked rather innocently, "What will happen after my baby is born?" The nurse looked at me blankly, as if she were confused and didn't quite understand the meaning of my question. "Why, nothing," she replied. "You will just go home and take care of your baby." She wasn't being arrogant. She just couldn't imagine what I was getting at. I pressed further. "Well, how do I do that—take care of my baby?" "Let's not go into that now," she responded. "Why don't we save that discussion for our last session?" I agreed but inwardly I was dissatisfied with her reply. We never did get to the promised discussion of postpartum recovery. We spent our six weeks handling plastic replicas of cervixes and pelvic bones at various points in dilation. We sighed, panted, puffed, and hissed, making all the required sounds of prepared childbirth. We tried to transcend our imaginary labor pains while lying on our imaginary beaches—"breathing and relaxing, breathing and relaxing." We saw a movie of a pink-faced, red-haired mother delivering her baby under a white sheet. We spent weeks preparing for delivery, which is almost always less than a day's time—sometimes simply a few hours. But we learned nothing about the time that follows. Doesn't that sound rather ludicrous to you?

The truth is, I had heard whispers about postpartum depression, the infamous "baby blues," and I was determined not to have them. After all, for most of my adult life I had been healthy, active, and careful about my diet. I was a survivor. Besides, how much trouble could a little baby be?

All of my precautions proved to be of no avail, for exactly seventy-two hours after the birth of my little girl, I was sitting in the corner of my bed trembling uncontrollably. I cried for four solid hours, and I didn't know why. I thought I was having a nervous breakdown. What I had was a case of the "blues," and that was just the beginning.

I returned to work at my studio precisely four weeks after my delivery. After all my proselytizing about the vital role of exercise in prenatal and postpartum care, I felt I had to be the shining example to my students. I bundled up my tiny daughter in a corduroy "Snugli," and off we went to work. While I instructed my classes, I wheeled her about in a collapsible stroller. She became my "assistant." I breast-fed her in the dressing room, and she napped on the exercise mats. Soon the population of new moms and babies grew to such a proportion that the studio owner hired a baby-sitter. There I was, teaching class amidst a chorus of wailing babies.

Each day was a little different, but I knew something was wrong. There was a sense of tension brewing as I carefully adjusted a leg or asked a back to straighten or a stomach to flatten in class. I felt as if I woke up each morning and deliberately threw myself totally into my work to avoid having to look directly at the emotional confusion of my life. Every postpartum mother seemed to be terrified of this emotional confrontation in very much the same way. They couldn't say how they really felt. I myself was afraid. I felt alienated from my husband, my family, my friends. Was it abnormal to feel like this? Was it lack of sleep that was causing me to function in a zombie-like fashion, afraid to feel anything lest I burst into tears?

Finally the walls of silence began to break down. The new mothers began to talk to me and I to them. We were not talking about our babies anymore but about ourselves. Our feelings were mutual. We loved our babies but we certainly wouldn't have minded if they disappeared for a few hours or for an entire evening, for that matter. We'd give a few years of life for a single-night's sleep—and we all felt twinges of guilt for feeling this way. We all felt tired, angry, alone, and disillusioned. We also discovered that there was some unwritten law for new mothers. Never tell anyone your true feelings about this time—especially not a pregnant woman! God forbid we spoil her "blooming." Why all this secrecy? Talking was the one thing that made us feel alive again. It was so good to know that we weren't going mad.

We, the women of the eighties, are rather fortunate in one aspect. Today there is a greater wealth of knowledge on the subject of pregnancy and childbirth than there ever was before. We (women between the ages of twenty-five and forty), who are the children of the last "baby boom," which succeeded World War II and the Korean War, have matured and are parenting the present "boom." Thanks to pioneers like Elisabeth Bing, Dr. Leboyer, and Dr. Lamaze, women no longer fear labor pain, isolation in childbirth, or the sterile hospital environment that our mothers may have faced thirty or forty years ago. Now there is information on becoming pregnant and staying pregnant, on diverse methods of natural childbirth, and on both exercise and nutrition during pregnancy. However, if there is any information on postpartum recovery in books about childbirth, it is usually dismissed in a paragraph or two. If you are lucky, you may find a single chapter on the postpartum period. It is true that there is invaluable information contained in these books, and all women should avail themselves of this vital information to make their pregnancies and deliveries as rewarding as possible. But why, I ask, isn't the same kind of information available to the woman in the midst of postpartum recovery?

As I researched this question, I came up with a few answers. Historically, women's issues have been ignored. Male researchers traditionally have not been interested in women's health problems, so the research just doesn't get properly funded and as a result just doesn't get done.

For example, the New York Academy of Medicine library, which is representative of all good medical libraries, has at this writing in its BRS-MESH bank (BRS-MESH is an on-line data base related to the Medline data base, which contains virtually all available medical information worldwide) only eighty-eight references to postpartum depression in the period 1966–1982. This information includes articles from noted medical journals, films, doctoral dissertations from universities, and excerpts from some of the more obscure medical periodicals.

While this may sound like a wealth of material, upon further investigation I found that many of these articles were not directly concerned with postpartum depression. Some merely contained the phrase "postpartum depression," or "puerperium," the medical term for the period immediately following childbirth. These studies encompassed worldwide information, but because they were specifically geared to the medical population, they were often totally incomprehensible to the lay person. This means that in the sixteen-year period between 1966 and 1982, there were only eighty-eight instances in which the medical profession investigated postpartum depression or even referred to it. In comparison to other medical problems, such as ulcers or migraine headaches, to which there are literally thousands of references in medical journals and from which only a small portion of our population suffers, postpartum recovery is poorly documented. And because of the highly technical language and the nature of this material, it is unavailable to the average woman.

It may be advisable at this point in my discussion to define depression. Unfortunately, depression has come to be known by its symptoms and not by what it actually is. Depression is certainly not a disease in the sense that a viral disease, for example, is. Essentially, depression is a disorder, a disorder slightly different from others in that it involves both physical and psychological factors. Physically, depression is a manifestation of chemical imbalances in the body. Psychologically, it may represent a significant life change or crisis point in the life of an individual. Depression can be normal, as a natural result of a specific life situation, or pathological, but in either case it is fundamentally marked by a decrease in functional activity and a feeling of inadequacy. Higher animals such as monkeys and dogs also exhibit elements of depressive behavior. Though they do not possess sufficient intelligence to experience inadequacy, their physical activities will diminish in very much the same way a depressed human's will.

Postpartum depression is unique. It has a pattern of symptoms and environmental overlays that sets it apart from other forms of depression. It is also peculiar in that, since almost every childbearing woman experiences it, it is taken out of the realm of pathology and placed in the realm of normal life experiences. In the *Dissertion Abstracts International*,[1] it was reported that both the mothers of newborn infants and the mothers of eighteen-month-old infants are significantly more depressed than childless women. The authors concluded from this study that the specific symptoms of postpartum depression are directly associated with becoming a mother and not just with being female, a notion that has been held previously. In addition, some form of stress—marital, financial, or social—has been presented as a major contributor to postpartum depression. Technically, stress is defined as nervous tension. It may be physical, as in sickness, or emotional, as in the loss of a job, and it may also be conscious or unconscious, since we are often unaware of the initial signs of stress. Stress may be temporary or it may be chronic—stress accumulating in a continuing situation. Whatever tensions occur in our lives, the most important thing is how we deal with them. Because motherhood embodies biological, emotional, and social tensions, it is a potentially stressful point in the lives of women.

To understand better why there has been so little research on this significant life issue, perhaps it would be useful to look at how postpartum depression has been viewed historically. The women's issues which have been addressed most recently are those in which men feel they play an active role. Issues such as sex, pregnancy, and childbirth have always represented hallmarks in a man's life. Signs of male fertility are heralded in all cultures. Other topics, such as menstruation, breast cancer, or postpartum depression (though they have been discussed briefly), have been slower to surface because they are traditionally associated with purely female functions. Also, until this century, women's complaints have not been considered vital, because of a traditionally male-dominated world.

When a male attained sexual maturity in ancient or primitive cultures, the event was marked with joy and celebration. When a woman reached the corresponding maturity, with the menarche (initial menstruation), she was often cast out from her tribe, buried waist deep in sand, or made to endure some other unspeakable mental or physical torture. Often a women's hands were bound behind her back in the belief that if she touched a living thing during this time it would die. This tendency still prevails, though inconspicuously. I remember the accompanist for my ballet classes, a spunky eighty-four-year-old woman, once telling me that when she had had her period she had never touched flowers for fear they would wilt!

This same kind of morbidity and fear seems historically to

have shrouded the postpartum period. Hippocrates, the fourth-century B.C. Greek medical writer, observed that the postpartum phenomenon was a kind of "madness" caused by excessive bloodflow to the brain. He felt that the onset of lactation brought about the despair and delirium. The same notion was held by mid-nineteenth-century physicians, who termed postpartum depression "milk fever." In the Middle Ages it was believed that evil demons occupied a new mother's body. The forms of exorcism to rid her of demons were often so severe that the new mother, in a crazed emotional state, would strangle her own child—making infanticide the most common form of murder during this period. The Victorians also regarded postpartum as a time of mystery. The upper-class postpartum mother was in her "confinement" from her last trimester of pregnancy until about eight weeks postpartum. During this time, she was not allowed to leave her bed or accept visitors, usually had her newborn in the care of a wet nurse, and was said to have a case of the "vapors"—the Victorian term for all female disturbances. She often was not seen in public again until her baby was at least six months old.

The Freudians were not too kind to postpartum mothers, either. They dismissed completely the idea that postpartum depression had any physical aspects. Freud believed that postpartum depression was a neurosis produced by unresolved oedipal conflicts. The new mother, in a sense, hated her own mother and thus refused to accept her new role, with which she identified her maternal parent.

Now the pendulum has swung in the opposite direction. Today theorists believe that postpartum depression is largely physical, the result of tremendous hormonal fluctuations. Of course, there are instances in which either the physical or emotional aspect will dominate. There are documented cases of women suffering from postpartum depression who are not biological mothers but adoptive mothers. Obviously, their condition is largely psychological. The point is, however, that no matter what the cause, postpartum depression is real and it can be very painful. *Yet, with the right information and with loving support, it can be overcome.*

Postpartum depression is an area about which very little is known. And though there are women who never experience any symptoms of postpartum depression, from my research it appears that more than half of new mothers do. Instances of postpartum depression in first-time mothers range from 60 to 85 percent, with statistics slightly higher for women having a second child. These statistics include all degrees of depression, ranging from very mild depression to clinical depression, which requires psychiatric intervention.

Women experiencing postpartum depression are extremely vulnerable. Statistics demonstrate with great clarity that you are four to five times more likely to develop a psychological disorder during the first three months of motherhood than at any other point in your life. In addition, the first six months of postpartum make you more predisposed to emotional difficulties than other members of the female population.

Women as a group are far more prone to the symptoms of depression than are men—a staggering six times more susceptible! There is research available that indicates that these statistics may be unreliable, as men simply hide their depression better than women. This theory states that men traditionally associate emotional disorders with weakness and thus will not go for treatment, lest they expose themselves. If men don't appear in treatment as often as women do, it is assumed that they do not experience depression as often. This theory, of course, has yet to be confirmed.

The realities of the postpartum experience may sound alarming to you and, in a way, they are alarming. However, the truth is that 95 percent of women recover from postpartum depression, and the remaining 3 to 5 percent accounts for women who previously showed signs of mental imbalance. The real dilemma is that most women go into postpartum recovery as if into the wilderness. They carry no provisions—only a little common sense and some stale advice. That is not enough.

Whether or not you suffer from postpartum depression, this book can do several things for you as a new mother. And it is a different kind of new-mother's book. It is written by postpartum mothers. You will not learn how to change a diaper, sterilize a bottle, or take a temperature. You will certainly not be told that, since you will get over this period soon enough, you might as well forget about it. But you will learn several new things. First, you will learn that you are not alone—that your feelings after childbirth are universal. You will also find out how to recognize the symptoms of depression and get advice on how to find help. Second, you will learn about your body—why you look the way you do and what you can do about it. Carefully planned nutrition and exercise programs are included here; I have also added a playtime section on creative exercises you and your baby can share. You will learn how to improve your body image—what to do to become the attractive woman you were before childbirth. Third, you will learn about the responsibilities of both the working mother and the "unsalaried" working mother. And, fourth, you will learn about that new love triangle—you, your husband, and your baby.

But most important, you will learn how to cope and how to make your postpartum recovery the most conducive to your physical and emotional well-being. The past and present myths that surround new motherhood must be erased and replaced with pertinent information. This book is for all women of childbearing age, especially those pregnant at present or those considering starting a family. It is also addressed to your husbands, so they can create a more supportive environment for your new family.

The Complete Postpartum Guide is a deeply personal book, a consciousness-raising book—a book about our potential growth as mothers, as women, and as people in society. It is only when we can realize this potential that we can find strength in ourselves and in our new families.

═══1═══

"What Are the 'Baby Blues'?"
Your Emotions

"What Will Life Be Like?"
Feelings During Pregnancy

Almost all of us have expectations of motherhood. Recent literature and the media have emphasized to us the tremendous beauty of both pregnancy and childbirth. Many women plan and enjoy their pregnancies.

However, no woman I have interviewed has greeted the discovery of her pregnancy without some reservation. As one woman reported,

> *I don't know what was wrong with me. Here I was thirty-four years old. My husband and I had planned this baby. We had waited for just the right time and yet I was so confused. Had I made a mistake? I felt so guilty. Here was a time when I should have been so grateful and all I was was dismayed.*

Although most of us recover from these early feelings of ambivalence and are happy to announce the news, there still lingers, in the most perfect of circumstances, feelings of insecurity and doubt. I myself remember sitting on the edge of my bed repeating over and over, "I'm pregnant. I'm really pregnant." I walked over to my dresser and stared into the mirror. Had I changed? Was "I" still there?

Your feelings about your pregnant state are likely to change. Your initial symptoms will wear off and so will most of the initial anxieties (though never completely), and one morning you will awaken to find that you are no longer "gagging" down breakfast or falling asleep at the dinner table. You gaze into that same mirror and there is that adorable face, though slightly rounder, of course, all rosy and smooth. Your eyes are glistening and your hair is thick and shiny. So what if you have a protruding stomach—you have full, voluptuous breasts to match. Besides, you are expected to look that way. And you gradually stroll down the path of euphoria.

I was never happier than during my first pregnancy. I had no cares. I had nothing to concentrate on other than my baby. During my lunch hour, when I usually went shopping, I had someone else to shop for. I would rummage through the racks of blues and pinks and yellows. I could eat what I wanted. I could even take a little nap at work without feeling guilty. If I didn't want to go to a certain party, I could just say that I was a little worn out and they would understand.

I felt like a statue, like I should be immortalized in a park somewhere. There I would be forever—motherhood in all of her glory.

There are many advantages to pregnancy other than the obvious. Our culture respects pregnancy—makes allowances for it. Some women may not have had good relationships with their own mothers and may have been rebellious during their adolescence. However, even if this has been the case, many mothers and daughters call a temporary truce during pregnancy and begin to develop a close relationship. Motherhood is

something your mother understands. There is immediate identification. Your employer and coworkers understand, too. They
cover for you when you are "under the weather" and certainly
don't squawk if you are thirty minutes late coming back from
an appointment with your obstetrician. You may even get a
seat on the bus for once! Your husband, too, is unusually attentive. When you walk down the street together, people look at
you differently, as if they are saying, "Aren't they wonderful?
They are having a baby."

The "doll-babies" of our childhood become more and
more real to us as we stop on the street and peek into newly
decorated prams. "Soon, I will have one too," we think. We
stand polishing the dining-room table one day, stare out the
window, and think, "What's it really going to be like—having a
baby? What will I do? Will I ever be the same?"

The answer, sadly yet joyfully, is no. You will not be the
same. Pregnancy and childbirth are viewed by many new
mothers as an end. But, in fact, they are only the beginning.
Your life will change when you have a baby, and the adjustments you will need to make as a result of this change will be
difficult and confusing. The way you feel about yourself during the postpartum period is often unanticipated during the
joyful moments of pregnancy. To help you understand better
the many-layered feelings of postpartum recovery, let's go on
to the next section and discover how many postpartum mothers
do feel.

"DOES EVERYONE FEEL THE WAY I DO?"

*I feel as if I am empty now. I'm somehow only half the
person I was. I cry a lot now and am so afraid of doing
something wrong. Yet my baby is so wonderful. I actually
have a new respect for myself now that I am a mother.*

The first thing I want to emphasize is that postpartum
depression is absolutely normal and that almost all mothers are

plagued with the same kind of ambivalent feelings that this young mother expressed. The time following the birth of a child is a crisis point in your life and requires special adjustments.

During the last three months of pregnancy, your body is literally flooded with hormones. These hormones make you relaxed and complacent, able to tolerate a previously unhandled amount of stress. During this time you appear to be ecstatic with joy. Nothing bothers you. You become exuberantly happy—almost "giddy," "silly," or "drunk."

Within hours of childbirth, however, these hormones taper off a dramatic 40 percent. The effect of that hormonal change can make you feel as if you had just fallen off a cliff. Your emotions are spiraling you into a truly chaotic state of mind. It is similar to having been addicted to barbiturates for nine months and subsequently suffering the symptoms of withdrawal. The ecstasy you may feel during late pregnancy and childbirth can be replaced by anger, deep sadness, and fear. These can be purely endrogenous reactions, symptoms produced by severe chemical changes, but they do have psychological overlays.

By current medical definition, postpartum depression progresses through roughly three stages: 1) the first ten days after delivery; 2) the next three months; 3) the final three months, which culminate with your child's six-month birthday. This is an extremely conservative view and, most medical experts agree, very incomplete. In the University of Michigan study that I cited earlier, documented results showed that there was no significant difference between the depression levels in the mothers of newborns and the depression levels of the mothers of eighteen-month-old children. This indicates that the depression levels of the women tested did not drastically decline after the traditional six-month period, as had previously been theorized.[1]

Unfortunately, there has been very limited research in this area to validate completely the existence of postpartum depression, by this pure definition, and beyond these narrow bound-aries. There are, however, innumerable indications that post-partum recovery can extend, to the outermost point, into your child's second year. One such study, presented in London's *Psychological Medicine* journal in 1976,[2] indicated a signifi-cant incidence of psychotic episodes during the tenth and twenty-fourth month after delivery, and also well into the fourth year after birth. This study is further validated in Ox-ford's *Journal of Child Psychology and Psychiatry*, which re-ports significant depression statistics, of between 26 and 40 per-cent, in mothers of preschool children.[3] The symptomatology of this later period does, of course, need further clarification, in order to be included in this broader definition of postpartum recovery.

I personally feel that the first year after your child's birth is crucial to your emotional development. That is why I have chosen to discuss postpartum recovery within the framework of that first year. The first six months of this period will be more representative of the physical, or hormonal, reactions associat-ed with postpartum depression, while the latter six months will reflect more the situational, or cultural, aspects of mothering. This is not to say that both the physical and emotional aspects will not be present throughout that entire year, but that the balance will differ.

No matter how well prepared you may feel before deliv-ery, the continual demands of a new infant are almost always a shock. In the most basic sense, your life changes when you have a baby, and this essential concept is not readily accepted by most women. It must be learned within the confines of that first year.

The initial stage of postpartum depression, the first ten days after delivery, is the most conspicuous. It is here that two thirds of the psychotic episodes occur. It is marked by incessant crying, temper tantrums, and withdrawal. You may have thoughts of death and abandonment, unfounded phobias, or impulses about leaving the house or injuring the baby. You may hate yourself, your husband, or your child. A study in the December 1981 issue of the *Journal of Affective Disorders*[4] reported on eighty-one postpartum women who had been asked to rate their mood on a scale of emotions which included happiness, depression, tears, anxiety, irritability, and lability (vulnerability). Scores from the fifth postpartum day indicated a sharp rise in depression, tears, and lability. In the 1979 *Women and Health* journal,[5] early postpartum symptoms reported included tiredness, insomnia, irritability, and unprecipitated episodal crying.

Many postpartum mothers experience this extreme tearfulness and vulnerability during their first weeks of puerperium. You may begin to cry for no apparent reason. I remember beginning to weep in the middle of a telephone conversation. My caller only wanted to congratulate me on the birth of my baby, yet I began to cry so uncontrollably that I had to end our call. On another occasion, my grandmother, who was taking care of me during this time, had prepared a soft-boiled egg for my breakfast; I saw the egg and how easily it cracked, and suddenly I began to weep. I had recognized in this soft-boiled egg the softness and vulnerability of my own emotional state.

Many women have similar reactions:

I was watching a commercial and I suddenly began to cry. The commercial wasn't sad but it certainly touched a nerve. I cried for three solid hours.

Other women report incidences of irritability or extreme hostility:

My husband had cooked dinner and had burnt the carrots. I began to scream so loud that my whole body began to shake. I was hysterical with anger. I locked myself in the bathroom and stayed there terrified of what I might do if I came out.

After this initial postpartum stage, these symptoms do not pick up and disappear, as some professionals will have you believe. The fatigue, crying, temper tantrums, and feelings of hopelessness will follow you well into your third month of postpartum. Once your baby begins to sleep more regularly, you can hope for a reprieve. This usually happens four to five months after delivery. Merely by virtue of getting more recuperative sleep, you will begin to feel more in control. By your child's six-month birthday, you will feel a sudden sense of relief. Your baby's demands will significantly drop. The feeling of relief, however, is often temporary, for the new mother begins to be more influenced by environmental factors. The "time-energy crunch" sets in. If a woman hasn't already gone back to work, she begins to wonder about time management in general. What is she going to do about baby-sitters, child-care centers, and the housework? Even if the new mother makes a decision not to return to her job or career, she often will consider going back to school or engaging in some other creative outside activity at this six-month point. Essentially, after six months of absorption with her child, the average woman suddenly realizes, if she hasn't already, that she wants to do more than be a mother. She wants to do something for herself, and this decision is highly seasoned with complications. Since women, as opposed to men, are usually burdened the most with the arrangements of both mothering and outside interests, the positive decision to "rejoin the world" is often in itself a source of continuing stress for the new mother. A frequent result is frustration, as the new mother tries to accomplish everything and finds out that she can't.

When I come home from work, I'm exhausted. My daughter is squealing for her dinner and the breakfast dishes are still in the sink. My day begins at six A.M. and sometimes doesn't end until midnight. Even though I enjoy my daughter and my career, I sometimes wonder if it's all worth it.

After you emerge from that initial six-month "twilight-zone" period of parenting, you finally realize that being a mother is a total commitment and that there is often no absolute solution to balancing your own interests and the interests of your family. When this happens, I find that implementing the solution of "no solution" is very effective. This means accepting the fact that there may be no immediate way to resolve your predicament. Though there are many practical methods of coping with the adjustments of new motherhood, which I will describe in the chapters to come, simply by facing the reality of "no solution" you can save yourself from being totally unfair to yourself. Remember—you are a human, not a machine.

Perhaps one of the most clearly confirmed theories about postpartum depression is that any unresolved emotional conflicts you may have had before or during your pregnancy are bound to surface and explode with intensity during this time. Women who have had a history of depression are likely to suffer in the postpartum period.

The 1978 issue of *Psychoanalytical Study of the Child*[6] states that many cases of postpartum depression are symptomatic of underlying predisturbances. In the *Dissertation Abstracts International*[7] premenstrual tension is cited as the best indicator of postpartum depression. Oxford's *Journal of Psychosomatic Research*[8] confirmed the hypothesis that the highest levels of depression during pregnancy predicted the highest levels of depression during puerperium. At the annual meeting of the American College of Obstetricians and Gynecologists, as reported in the *Medical World News*,[9] experts also confirmed that postpartum psychosis is directly reflective of underlying psychological problems.

Thus, becoming significantly depressed during postpartum recovery may not be coincidental. One mother confided:

> *I was always irritable right before my period. During postpartum, I became particularly edgy. I couldn't stand*

*having anything out of place and with a new baby that
was pretty near impossible.*

Women who experience depression in general tend to be
perfectionists and, as a result, often feel inadequate when unable to achieve their unrealistic expectations. This inadequacy
tends to surface at life-crisis points, which include postpartum
recovery.

This information should not frighten you, but it will in-
form mothers who have had a tendency toward depression previously and will warn new mothers. The stress of new motherhood can aggravate an emotional condition. On the positive
side, being prepared and recognizing the symptoms of depression may force you into dealing with emotional issues that you
may have previously avoided.

The theory that postpartum depression can be predicted
has also been documented. There are studies to indicate that
certain personality types and life situations are more conducive
to postpartum depression than others. In the *Journal of Obstetrics and Gynecology*,[10] an experiment was reported that was
conducted to determine women at risk for what was termed
PED, postpartum emotional disorder. Six factors were shown to
be causal in determining cases of severe postpartum depression.

All of these factors—with one exception, which I will explain later—concern the postpartum mother's immediate relationships: specifically, the new mother's relationship with her
husband and with her new baby. Feeling unloved by her husband was the most predictive factor determining severe postpartum depression, followed closely by having an undesired
pregnancy. Other predictive factors included being single or
separated from her husband, having an unplanned pregnancy,
or having marital problems in general.

From this study, it appears that both a woman's relationship with her husband and her feelings about her pregnancy
can be significant in determining her emotional state following
childbirth. This information contradicts a still rather widely
held notion that the birth of a child can improve a bad mar-

riage. It does not. In a good marriage, the birth of a child can pose difficulties; in a bad marriage, the birth of a child can be impossible to deal with. It is also very important for a woman to want her pregnancy. The wide availability of a variety of birth-control methods can truly allow every couple to plan their family rather than simply have a family "happen to them."

Another predictive factor determined by this study was having a history of postpartum depression. This factor confirms the theory I previously discussed, which states that postpartum depression does not simply occur. It is often preceded by other depressive episodes, during other periods of life crises.

One study, in the *British Journal of Medical Psychology*,[11] indicated that women who rated high on hostility and loss-of-control in screening, given during the thirty-sixth week of their pregnancy, also rated high in these when screened postnatally. That is, women who felt that they were not in control of their lives tended to develop more pronounced cases of postpartum depression. Also, the results of this study showed that younger women seemed to be more susceptible than older women.

Further, this study validates my previously stated correlation between postpartum depression and feelings of inadequacy. Perhaps women who are essentially insecure and who may truly feel that their lives are controlled by others, as well as younger women who may not have developed the inner confidence of life experience, may be more susceptible to developing pronounced cases of postpartum depression.

Another study, involving first-time-parent couples, which was conducted at the University of Michigan, concluded that: 1) husbands were generally not depressed during puerperium, 2) wives who were depressed during pregnancy were often depressed postnatally.[12] This study also stated, "The findings suggest that postpartum depression can be predicted. Pregnant women should be encouraged to report any signs of emotional distress and professionals should be educated to recognize these signs as possible predictors of difficulty after birth."

The findings of this study cannot be overstated. The fact is that many pregnant women are not encouraged to report their emotional discomfort. Some obstetricians have difficulty enduring their patients' discussion of physical complaints. In addition, there are so few screening devices available for detecting potential puerperial depression that it often is undiscovered until a woman has a pronounced psychotic episode. This is sad, because many of these episodes can be prevented with the proper psychiatric intervention and early detection. As a pregnant woman can be determined a physical risk through prenatal biological screenings, she should likewise be given a standard prenatal-depression screening to determine if she has any predisposing factors for postpartum depression. If it is determined that she is at risk in this area, she should be given the appropriate psychological treatment during her pregnancy so that the potential stress of her postpartum period may be alleviated.

In another University of Michigan study, ninety-one new mothers reported a 52 percent prevalence of depression.[13] Causes included: 1) hostile attitudes toward mother figures; 2) biological and situational stress; 3) feelings of inwardly turned aggression accompanied by a sense of hopelessness.

Maggie Scarf, in her enlightening book on depression, *Unfinished Business*, illustrates the conclusions of this Michigan study. The triad of previously stated causal factors is apparent in Scarf's presentation of "Laurie," a postpartum mother. During an interview, Laurie says:

> I wanted to do it all. I wanted to do everything as far as the children were concerned . . . but I also wanted my freedom. So there I was finally, working hard to have it both ways. And I was finding it—oh, it was getting close to impossible. I was feeling so bad, as if I couldn't bear the sight of another day, another morning. Each time I thought I wouldn't get through this one; that I couldn't make it, couldn't bear it, couldn't go on.[14]

Laurie was the mother of two children and also taught social work. She was a perfectionist. She wanted everything.

She began to resent her role as a mother, became overwhelmed by stress, and began to blame herself because she was unable to manage her life in the manner she expected. This is not an unusual situation. It is, in fact, symptomatic of many cases of postpartum depression. However, further research needs to be conducted and findings confirmed so that we can understand better the nature of postpartum depression. The Michigan study I just described reiterates this concern: "A broad approach in understanding and treating postpartum depression is indicated as essential."[15]

There have been further studies to both cite new and reaffirm the previously mentioned causal factors in postpartum depression.

In a recent issue of the Oxford *Journal of Child Psychology and Psychiatry*,[16] it is stated that women who have comparatively fewer material and social resources tend to be more depressed after delivery than those with access to these resources. It is also felt that the care of children is a potent stress factor in and of itself. Another University of Michigan study pointed to the combined interaction of three factors predicting postpartum depression. These three factors were: 1) premenstrual tension; 2) recent life stress; 3) marital adjustment.[17]

Though the relationship of both premenstrual tension and marital adjustment regarding postpartum depression have been previously emphasized, when these two factors are coupled with recent life stress, this combination becomes an even more critical indicator of potential postpartum difficulties. Life stress, which I will refer to in later chapters, even as an isolated causal factor, can be significant in determining a new mother's postpartum reaction. Stress, as I have described earlier, is nervous tension generally triggered by outside circumstances. Stress can be produced by a variety of life situations, and reactions to stress vary with individuals. Both pregnant women and postpartum mothers need to be aware of the events in their lives which are potential stress producers. Profoundly significant stress signals would, of course, be death in the immediate family, divorce, or severe illness of a loved one. If these circumstances parallel the birth of your child, you should be prepared for a temporary emotional imbalance. However, there are also some less significant life events that, due to their "insignificance," tend to be ignored by many new mothers as potential causes for emotional tension. Fairly common events—such as moving to a new home, you or your husband taking on new responsibilities at work, or taking an extended trip—are all relatively stress-producing. Both the pregnant women and the postpartum mother need to pace their lives to avoid the inevitable emotional drain. If, for example, you need to relocate to a new city due to professional obligations, try to do so at least six months before your baby's arrival. Preparation and awareness of the stress that often accompanies major life adjustments can help you to cope more efficiently with your postpartum recovery.

Whatever other emotional aspects may be present, depression in women tends to revolve around one pervading issue: the sense of loss. During our lifetimes we become attached to many things—our homes, our parents, our friends, our spouses, our careers—but, more importantly, we become attached to ourselves in relationship to these things. Yes, we actually become attached to our own identities. Any severance of the images we hold of ourselves can bring on inward conflict. We all know the trauma of moving away from home or breaking up with a long-term boyfriend. But these separations are often necessary to the establishment of self. Somewhere along the journey to maturity, we find our *self,* and although we may actively dislike parts of that self, we cling to it because it belongs to us. As I will describe later, during postpartum depression many images a woman may have previously held about herself seem to disappear.

It has been shown statistically that men do not become depressed over this "loss of self" in relation to attachment issues—at least not in the same manner that women do. Men are more caught up in "success" and "making it." A man's sense of self is more often measured in terms of achievement rather than in terms of relationships. A large part of this is culturally induced. A woman's sense of self is likely to be more focused on personal issues than is a man's.

The cumulative emotional effect of new parenthood probably represents the greatest single period of loss in your life. It seems as if everything has changed. If you worked, more than likely you have left your job, at least temporarily. Your baby has left the confines of your body. You've even lost the shape and strength of your body. Most significantly, though, you can feel as if you've lost yourself.

The period of adolescence, in a sense, is a parallel to postpartum depression. It too is a time of tremendous hormonal changes accompanied by emotional stress. Our bodies grow and mature: we change from little girls to sexual women. Often adolescents will turn on their parents in a painful attempt to separate themselves from childhood and establish themselves as adults. Interesting, too, is that teenage pregnancy in unmarried girls is often correlated with depression. It is as if the young girl, unable to break fully from her parents, forms another union with her baby, in an effort to obtain the love which she can no longer ask from her mother and father.

The truth is that most of us make it to adulthood with a few scratches, to be sure, but without major complications. Yet the period of adolescence is felt keenly by most people. For many women the separation from parents during growth from adolescence to maturity can be complicated. In the past, and often now, parents expect their daughters to be virginal. The growth to sexual maturity and independence for a young woman can be more painful than for a young man. And often in the process, adolescents feel hostile toward parents, as well as themselves, precisely because they are so dependent upon them for emotional support. The same kind of growth process takes place during postpartum recovery. Though the emotions of being a new mother may be painful, they prepare us physically and psychologically for the responsibilities of motherhood. Like adolescence, postpartum depression has a beginning, a middle, and, fortunately, an end. Also, it is important to note that mothering does not have to be an end in itself. The basic skills and emotional adjustments which women struggle with in that first year are a progressive adventure in learning about themselves as well as their children.

An answer to my initial question, "Does everyone feel the way I do?" is yes: almost all new mothers experience stress and depression as a result of childbirth.

On Being a Mother:
Images and Cultural Attitudes

Though we've established that postpartum depression is both physical and psychological in nature, it is also culturally based. Many sociologists and psychologists believe that Western society's glorification of motherhood sets up insecurity and guilt in women who may not feel adequate to fulfill the requirements of motherhood.

> *I was determined to be the perfect mother—warm, loving. But when I tried to devote all my energy to my son, I started to become bored and resentful. My husband tried to console me, saying that I shouldn't let him run my life or that it was natural for me to want some time for myself, but I couldn't accept it. I loved my baby and I wanted to be with him, yet I seemed to expect so much from my relationship with him—much more than I expected from any other relationship.*

Mothers are susceptible to anger, fatigue, and irrationality just like everyone else. But that's not the picture that has been painted for us. We are brought up to believe that a mother is an all-loving, all-warm, all-giving creature; she has no self, no pride, no ambition. Her purpose in life is to guide, to comfort, to nourish. It's interesting that every woman I interviewed used the words "loving," "warm," "giving" when describing her image of a mother, yet not a single one felt that she was living up to that image.

A mother is someone who is always there. Someone you can always turn to when you need her. I'm always trying to live up to that image, but I never can.

One example I feel demonstrates this media phenomenon particularly well is what I will term the "Lucy syndrome." You remember Lucy. You can flick your television dial to various channels and watch her raise her children. I have to admire Lucy, for, in spite of her shortcomings, she managed to be pregnant and stand in front of millions of people in 1954. There was a real person underneath that tunic, not just stuffing. But Lucy was as antiseptic as the fifties. We, the new mothers of the eighties, grew up with Lucy. One minute we watched her complaining to Ethel about her tiredness and "blah" feeling. The next minute we watched those blue eyes of hers open in wild amazement upon discovering her pregnancy, and then we watched with anticipation as she perched on the edge of her modern Swedish couch, bedecked in blouson top, tightly fitted capris, and velvet slippers, waiting to tell Ricky.

To TV viewers, it appeared that Lucy's major problems during her pregnancy were decorating the nursery, trying to find enough room for all the toys she purchased, and, of course, that exasperating drive to the hospital. These events were made catastrophic, as only Lucy could make them. We laughed with her; it was entertaining.

When little Ricky did arrive, we barely noticed him, except for Lucy's occasional trips to the nursery to smile and coo. She was once again darting about in her designer dresses and carefully coiffed hair. She was never housebound with a sick child. If she had something really important to do, there was always the reliable Mrs. Trumble to babysit on the spur of the moment. Lucy didn't have the baby blues.

So, in the last decades, it seemed to would-be mothers that babies would ornament their lives. A baby would be kept tucked away like any other prized possession—to be displayed to private company or to curious passersby in the street.

Though there are unequaled joys to be experienced in mothering, most of what the media has presented to us is, at the least, an exaggeration and, at the most, a lie. Yet women continue to compete with a dream of motherhood that doesn't exist.

Despite the acknowledged discrepancy between the myth and the reality of motherhood, our society does not present postpartum depression as being normal. It is viewed as neurotic, selfish, and just plain crazy. Yet experts have always known it existed. Society's condemnation of a new mother's confused emotional feelings can leave the average woman feeling highly inadequate. The following statement, taken from *Ourselves and Our Children,* by the Boston Women's Health Book Collective, says it all:

> I think that obstetricians and hospital staff are very negligent about talking about postpartum. It can be a long process of recovery. And if you haven't been led to see it as normal or likely, you feel somewhat panicked that you are going crazy. You have lost your strength and your clothes size and your sexual self image and maybe your job and your economic independence, your sense of adult community—and they call it the "baby blues." Instead they should help you, talk about diet and exercise and finding household and childcare help, and sharing with your husband. They don't want to scare you, so instead they leave you stranded.[18]

In order to overcome the pitfalls of misunderstanding the nature of the postpartum period, society first needs to recognize it as a phenomenon and to see postpartum depression as perfectly normal and not purely as a psychotic disorder. Postpartum depression is a phenomenon that exists for virtually every childbearing woman. It is not merely some "silliness" concocted by pampered Western women to attract attention.

There is incidence of postpartum depression throughout primitive cultures as well. *The Archives of General Psychiatry*[19] documented a study of East African postpartum mothers. It was demonstrated that close to 80 percent of the women studied experienced the symptoms of postpartum depression. Despite a different culture, the prevalence of postpartum depression was similar to that of more developed cultures.

Postpartum depression needs to be taken seriously. In mourning a loss through death, one is expected to be depressed and subsequently, over a reasonable amount of time, to recover. Postpartum depression deserves the same consideration. The most supportive act that members of the medical profession can perform is to let pregnant women know that postpartum depression is a real and an acceptable consequence of childbirth. An article in *Women and Health*[20] states that a woman's realization of the prevalence of postpartum depression may help both her and her husband accept and overcome it. The *West Virginia Medical Journal*[21] reiterates that indirectly by saying that, though psychiatric intervention is seldom required in cases of postpartum depression, it is necessary to allow the prospective parents to know that the symptomatology of postpartum depression is common and rarely indicative of mental illness.

Both the *Journal of Gynecology Nursing* and the *British Journal of Psychiatry* cite the significance of social pressure as contributing to the stress and confusion of postpartum depression:

> A theory is postulated to explain the potential that exists for cultural attitudes towards pregnancy to become precipitating agents in postpartum depressive syndrome. Changes in body proportion, public attitudes, and the social lives of expectant women are viewed primarily as negative experiences which result in the loss of self esteem.[22]

> ... overall findings indicate the importance of social stress in puerperal depression.[23]

What does society expect from its new mothers? Involvement, compliance—perhaps they expect us to be consumed by our new role. But most of all they expect us to be happy and grateful if we have a healthy baby. After all, what else could we possibly want? In a study conducted by social scientists,[24] results indicated that mothers who were not ready to respond to their child's every whim, who criticized their children when their behavior warranted it, and who sometimes felt that their own lives took priority over their children's were given a curious label. These women were termed as being "hostile mothers." They were labeled as hostile simply because they chose to create an atmosphere of independence in which to raise their children. They were not going to be maidservants; they were going to be people.

More interesting than this, however, is the follow-up research to this particular study. Scientists discovered, to their amazement, that during the twenty-five-year time span in which the children of this study became adults, the offspring of the so-called "hostile mothers" (the female offspring in particular) were more achieving and more independent, compared to the offspring of the nonhostile or less hostile mothers. The children of the "hostile mothers" were also better able to handle stress than the children of the nonhostile or less hostile mothers.

The study concluded that perhaps a certain amount of hostility was necessary to creating a responsible adult. Of course, I feel the term "hostile" is inappropriate here. These women were not hostile, in my opinion. They merely wanted to instill the value of self-reliance in their children. It may well be that our culture is so conditioned to the constant availability of mothering that the absence of it is simply viewed as rejection. Of course the terms "hostile" or "rejecting" are relative; these women were not rejecting their children—they were allowing them to find their own way. This attitude, in my opinion, is a far healthier one for families to flourish in than one in which the mother is on a twenty-four-hour alert. Essentially, the "hostile" mothers of this study ignored society and its precepts. They followed their own instincts, and they were proved successful mothers.

Besides being presented with this unrealistic view of motherhood culturally, the mothers in our generation are isolated from one another. When you don't have a "sounding board" whose experience echoes your own, you are even more predisposed to believing what the media will tell you. Many new mothers suffer terrible loneliness. Some are geographically far away from their own mothers, close relatives, and friends, and others just feel that their childless companions can't possibly understand what they are going through, and so they don't share their feelings.

True comradeship with other postpartum mothers has been cited as one of the chief antidotes for postpartum depression. It has even been effective in those cases where the depressive symptoms have been severe. In a unique and highly commendable program, conducted over seven years in a Vancouver clinic, former postpartum mothers are recognized by the clinic staff as the authorities on the problems of puerperial depression. In group-therapy sessions composed of new postpartum mothers, these women discuss how it feels to be depressed and how one can recover from depression. Informal sessions like this help to promote the idea that postpartum depression is a significant yet normal part of almost every childbearing woman's experience. In three American studies, interaction with postpartum mothers is cited as a preventive measure, when conducted with pregnant women, and as a therapeutic aid in cases of postpartum depression in new mothers.

Culturally, our expectations of motherhood and its reality have conflicted. We need to reexamine our traditional views in order to learn how to anticipate and cope with the postpartum experience. The only way we can do this adequately is to educate ourselves about the true conditions of mothering.

POSTPARTUM QUIZ: CRITERIA FOR INTERMEDIARY HELP

Though there is no one better able to judge your emotional state than your doctor, accompanied by a professional psychotherapist, here is a list of questions that may help you find out if you are in need of psychological assistance during your postpartum recovery. The test was prepared by Dr. Sujana Patibandla, M.D., a gynecologist at Roosevelt Hospital, New York, and by Dr. Robert Marc Fink, Ph.D., a clinical psychologist and the author of *Prepartum and Postpartum Depression: The Psychological Concomitants.*

Remember, when answering these questions, try to measure your comparative behavior. For example, if previous to your delivery you were content to eat three nutritious meals per day and now you find yourself unable to look at food, then there may be something wrong. But if you were a light eater, not wanting to eat now may not be so unusual. Also, though almost all of us have suffered from at least one (if not more) of the symptoms discussed below, it is the consistency and the combination of these symptoms that are likely to be an indication of serious difficulties. For example, simply being more irritable than usual may not be an indication of a serious problem in itself. You may have reason to be irritable. You may not be getting sufficient sleep during the postpartum period and as a result your nerves will naturally be on edge. However, if this irritability has been overwhelming and has persisted for several weeks, coupled with a generally depressed state of mind and feelings of inadequacy, then it is this combination of reactions that can be the indication of a depressive disorder. Take these points into consideration when answering the following questions.

Most, but not all, of the answers to the questions are self-explanatory. Therefore, after the more ambiguous questions I have included short explanations.

1. Are you feeling generally down, and has this state existed consistently for two weeks or more? Do you basically feel
that you don't care about anything anymore—that nothing
really matters? Do you literally wish you were dead or are you
continually thinking of suicide?

OR

Do you have more of a "seesaw" reaction—several days of
deep sadness followed by days of ecstasy with no apparent reason?

Question 1

If you can answer yes to either part of question 1, you may
be a victim of depression. Answer the questions that follow, to
try to form a clear picture of the depressive symptoms you may
be experiencing.

Note: Although passing feelings of depression and even
thoughts of suicide are common early in the postpartum period, these temporary feelings are not necessarily indications of
severe depression. To reiterate, it is the consistency and the
continual recurrence of these feelings that indicate a depressive
disorder warranting professional intervention, not simply the
feeling of depression itself. The "seesaw" reaction is medically
referred to as manic depression. It is an extremely common
form of depression and is characterized by the patient not having any "middle" feelings, such as tranquillity or satisfaction.
He is either ecstatic with joy or deeply depressed.

2. Have your eating habits changed dramatically—are
you undereating or overeating?
3. Have your sleep patterns altered? Do you have trouble
falling or staying asleep? Or are you sleeping incessantly without cause?

Questions 2 and 3

Changes in customary eating or sleeping patterns can be
indicative of a depressed state. Because you are a postpartum

mother, these patterns can be expected to change somewhat. However, if they become bizarre—if you are not eating at all or are overeating extremely, or if you are staying up all night or not being able to get out of bed in the morning, you may need special help.

4. Have your feelings about sexuality or sexual intercourse itself changed suddenly?

Question 4

Loss of libido is a common depressive symptom. Men experience impotence, and women the lack of orgasm. You can expect to be less interested in sexual activity during the early postpartum period simply because you are fatigued. However, if you begin to feel disgusted or embarrassed by your relationship with your husband to the point of fearing any affectionate display, then this denial or refusal of sexuality can indicate a deeply depressed condition. The reverse of this situation, manifesting itself in an obsession with sexual phenomena, can also indicate a loss of self-esteem; the person may involve herself with sexual matters and produce a guilt which in turn contributes to a feeling of worthlessness.

Note: Though many obstetricians advise against sexual intercourse during the first six weeks postpartum, sexual abstention for medical reasons does not indicate depression. It must also be noted that sexual intercourse is the only sexual activity being explicitly prohibited during this time, and that it is not being advised against because of its sexual nature. Obstetricians also advise against using tampons during the early postpartum period. Very simply, obstetricians are trying to prevent vaginal or pelvic infection, not sexual pleasure. Couples can continue to engage in other forms of sexual activity.

5. Are you having trouble concentrating?
6. Are you nervous and unable to sit still for any length of time?

Questions 5 and 6

The inability to concentrate or "sit still" is clinically known as hyperactive depression; it is characterized by a continual restlessness and the inability to finish any given project.

7. Are you more angry or irritable than usual?
8. Have you become intolerably pessimistic?
9. Do you feel worthless? Do you hate yourself?

Questions 7, 8, and 9

If you are more irritable or pessimistic than usual, or if you feel particularly worthless, then these feelings can be contributors to depression.

10. Do you feel guilty over past incidents that you can do nothing about?

Question 10

When you are obsessed with the past, you are setting yourself up to be a victim. The situation that produced the pain or guilt is over and cannot be altered in that context. If you are unable to rectify a past experience, it is sometimes best just to admit it to yourself rather than to dwell on a particular shortcoming.

11. Do you feel highly inadequate?
12. Do you have incessant crying spells?
13. Do you feel needy—constantly in need of self-assurance?

Questions 11, 12, and 13

Again, if these feelings of inadequacy or your crying spells are continual, then you may be in need of professional help.

14. Have you been suffering more than usual from physical complaints—severe headaches or backaches?

Question 14

There is abundant research to indicate the existence of psychosomatic illnesses. Emotional tension produces a wide range of physical complaints that cannot be treated in a traditional fashion.

15. Is your mouth constantly dry, with an accompanying bad taste?

Question 15

When a person is clinically depressed, the body's salt balance is altered. More salt than normal is retained in the cells of the body, resulting in water retention and subsequent mouth dryness. The mouth dryness can lead to an accompanying bad taste in the mouth. Theories vary on the physical causes for this water retention.

If you answer the first question affirmatively, and two or more of the subsequent questions affirmatively, you should consider a professional consultation with both your gynecologist and a trained psychotherapist.

IF YOU CHOOSE TO SEEK TREATMENT

There are several basic steps to take and there is information you need if you choose to seek treatment for postpartum depression. First, you must understand that depressive illnesses differ in individuals and thus require personalized treatment. Some postpartum depressive disorders can be treated chemically with progesterone and similar hormones, while other types require professional counseling. Other postpartum disorders may require a combination of these therapies or only one specific type of treatment.

The nature of severe postpartum depression needs to be properly diagnosed by a competent clinician. He will need to know whether your depression represents a lifelong pattern. He will need to ascertain your level of functioning—how well you are able to perform at work and at home with your child.

Finding a good psychotherapist is like finding any other professional. Lawyers, accountants, and secretaries are often referred by one's personal friends and acquaintances. The best place to start is with your gynecologist. If you are not pleased with the response to your problem, you have the option of seeking a second opinion. In any case, a professional psychiatrist or clinical psychologist is your best choice when seeking help for depressive illness. If you are still unable to find a suitable therapist, I would suggest calling a university-affiliated clinic. They will be able to provide you with a list of competent professionals in your vicinity.

If you do begin treatment and find you are not feeling better over a reasonable amount of time, it could be an indication that you need to reevaluate your situation and perhaps investigate other forms of treatment for your individual case.

I want to reiterate here that, though postpartum depressive disorders severe enough to warrant psychiatric intervention statistically occur in about 3 to 24 percent of the childbearing population, professional therapy is not ordinarily suggested as a natural succession to childbirth. The reason this percentage appears to be so high is that this research has not always been done with a normal population of women. Some has been conducted, without a control, with women who have had a history of psychiatric disorders and therefore have a higher potential for profoundly depressive symptoms postpartum, thus increasing the statistics in this area. When these statistics are correlated, they are apt to be biased because the experiments may not have been conducted with a group of women tested for parity. Three to 5 percent of all childbearing women is a more realistic percentage of women who will require psychiatric treatment for postpartum depression. The best rule is to stay in contact with your gynecologist. He will be best able to advise you about the natural as opposed to the extraordinary circumstances surrounding postpartum depression.

Almost every new mother will experience some degree of emotional discomfort during her postpartum recovery. Therefore, it is important for her to be able to distinguish between a normal postpartum reaction and what may be an indication of a depressive disorder. If a new mother understands the nature and symptoms of depression, she is better able to report these disturbances to her physicians and, if necessary, receive the appropriate treatment.

"What Can I Do?" A Practical Guide
to Coping with Your Feelings

Surprisingly, much of the advice I give is just plain common sense. Yet, it is often this very advice we choose to ignore. If it's possible, it's important to get household and child-care help— from a relative, friend, professional baby nurse, or housekeeper. The most common reaction to this suggestion is "Why do I need help? It's just going to be me and the baby." That's just the point. You and the baby are not enough. For at least the first two weeks, I recommend you have someone stay with you a minimum of eight hours a day, or until your husband gets home. Though baby nurses can be a godsend, unless you are bottle-feeding the baby or unless they opt for some of the housework, they can be useless. Let's face it. If you are breast-feeding your child, you have to be up in the middle of the night anyway. The only thing a baby nurse can do is bring the baby to you. My personal preference is to hire a housekeeper or arrange to have a relative clean the house. This way you can focus all your attention on the baby and not have to deal with the marketing or the laundry. Many housekeepers, if properly approached, will consent to take the baby outdoors for a stroll while you nap. Remember, your great-grandmother delivered her baby at home and was surrounded by her extended family during the first months. She didn't have to settle for struggle in solitude; why should you?

Next, get your husband properly involved. Granted, this takes time. Husbands are notorious for playing with infants while they are smiling, but when it comes to changing diapers, they hand the honors over to you. Though Chapter Six will go into this issue more fully, I want to say a few things here. Men, in general, have difficulty relating to infants. Why this is so has not been completely documented. Men, as a whole, tend to prefer older children, with whom they can communicate and with whom they can do things. However, the rewards for you and the baby from a committed husband are well worth it if you can be patient. Don't wait until your husband returns from work and immediately toss the baby into his arms and in your exhausted state shout, "Now, you take care of him!" This, however, is often the case, and the situation always creates unnecessary tension. Encourage your husband to bathe the baby and take him outdoors; most fathers enjoy parading their offspring.

With the growing trend toward breast-feeding, I encourage the purchase of a breast pump. Although some may contest this, I feel a breast pump can make all the difference to you in coping. Breast pumps can be operated either manually or electrically. The breast pump enables you to excrete and store your milk in the freezer.

If you can occasionally have your baby fed and cared for by someone else, you have options. I advocate taking at least one morning or one afternoon off during the work week to do something for yourself. You will feel less trapped and consequently less resentful of your new situation. You do not have to do anything special. If you are not too fatigued, go shopping or to the movies, or put your feet up and read a good novel or take that well-deserved nap. Remember, this is your own time. If you don't feel like being alone, go out with a friend. This may sound rather insignificant, but it sometimes can make all of the difference in the world during a period when you may feel isolated and resentful of your new responsibilities.

Communication is also important. Try not to lose touch with your friends. It is quite common among new mothers to get out of circulation because of time constraints:

> *We used to see Al and Judy almost every weekend. Now with the baby, I just don't have the freedom I used to. We can't take the baby anyplace and we can't be spontaneous. Everything has to be planned ahead of time—the baby-sitter and all. Judy would invite me somewhere and I'd have to cancel out. She seems to think that I am avoiding her or that I have a new life that doesn't include her anymore.*

It's true single friends and couples without children cannot possibly understand the complications that a child brings into a life. The best way to overcome this is to invite your friends into your home and let them see what goes on. After a few visits they will see the energy it takes to have an infant. They may even sympathize with you and offer their services as baby-sitters. It is especially important not to isolate yourself. I am not suggesting that you take up a complete social schedule immediately. That is simply not possible. Just try to maintain your friendships in a manner that is comfortable for all involved.

It is also extremely important to be with other new mothers. As I have stated earlier and cited from several studies, interaction with other postpartum mothers is essential in staving off the isolation that contributes to the symptoms of postpartum depression. The mutual support women in new-mothers' groups can offer each other is invaluable. The couples in your childbirth-preparation classes are good contacts for developing informal discussion groups. I know of several couples who met in prenatal classes and maintained active friendships for years after their children were born. There are new-mothers' groups forming throughout the country at Y's and other community organizations. If you are ambitious enough, you can start a new-mothers' or parenting group right in your living room. It takes nothing more than a few mothers (and new fathers) coming together and sharing their feelings. We all need camaraderie, especially at this crucial time.

Though I include an entire discussion on diet in Chapter Two, I want to say here that what you eat can also determine how you feel emotionally as well as physically. This is not the time to go out and try new things. Simple, nutritious food is what you need, not a smorgasbord. Keep away from the pizza parlors and the Indian curry kitchens. Anything too salty, too spicy, or too sour is going to be difficult to digest. If you are breast-feeding your baby, it's important for your baby, too, because all that you eat or drink filters eventually into your breast milk.

Proper exercise is never more essential than right now. Contrary to the traditional belief that exercise wears you out, it actually revitalizes you. Energy breeds energy, and vitality breeds vitality! I do not suggest that you go out and jog twelve miles tomorrow morning. But getting exercise is crucial to your health and sense of well-being. In Chapter Three, I have carefully outlined a sensible exercise program that you can begin right in your hospital bed. Some exercise can be harmful, but proper exercise is essential. A consistent fitness program during the postpartum period will not only give you back the shape and strength you once had, but will also contribute to a healthy mental attitude.

Last, enjoy your baby. Bringing a new and wonderful person into this world is truly a miracle. Nine months ago this little red-faced bundle sucking feverishly at your breast was nothing but a tiny microscopic seed. It grew and flourished inside you, then it left and crawled right into the center of your life. When you think about it, that's an unequaled experience!

"WHY DO I LOOK LIKE THIS?"
YOUR PHYSICAL SELF

YOUR BODY IMAGE

If we examine our lives as women, we can see several patterns of emotional crises. All the periods—the appearance of your menarche (initial menses), pregnancy and postpartum recovery, and menopause—are marked by extraordinary changes in body image. These significant changes in your body are almost always accompanied by corresponding emotional changes.

Recognizing that emotional and physical changes occur together is truly a departure from traditional Western theory, for we, as Western thinkers (as opposed to Eastern thinkers) are more accustomed to the concept of the separateness of mind and body rather than wholeness. In my last book, *Danceplay*, I gave a thorough explanation of mind/body duality as it applies to child development. However, it also very much applies to the various stages of both adolescent and adult growth and development.

For example, most women have rather despondent memories of adolescence. I, for one, waited for the appearance of my breasts with the usual concern. I am still waiting for their appearance. But being flat-chested at seventeen was much more devastating than it is now that I am in my thirties. Being a dancer, I acquired the traditional dancer's legs—muscular and well defined. In my teenage vanity, I interpreted this muscularity as bigness. So my chest was too flat and my legs were too big. I felt that my entire body had to be carefully hidden. For years I wore the biggest shirts and the baggiest pants I could find. In hiding my body so well, I also learned to bury parts of my personality. Many women I interviewed had experienced the same kind of emotional trauma during adolescence. It didn't matter what you looked like in reality. To yourself you felt physically inadequate, and these physical insecurities spilled over into your emotional life.

The same kind of "mind-body" pattern emerges during pregnancy and the postpartum period because for many these periods represent the greatest changes in body image for women. Men have no such counterpart in their lives and can often be unsympathetic. Let's face it. We are being given double messages. Eat well and stay healthy, but above all have the body of a beauty queen.

> *The first months of pregnancy were the most difficult for me. I didn't really look pregnant but I had gained ten pounds. I looked fat and felt fat. It really was depressing. When I finally began to look pregnant, it was a relief. I could finally blame my fatness on my pregnancy.*

The postpartum period, however, is even more depressing. You have nothing to blame your excess fat on except yourself. Along with your fat you have to make friends with your stretch marks, your milk-engorged breasts, your lost bladder control, your dry hair, and your bleeding gums.

> *I gained forty-eight pounds with my first pregnancy. I was so stupid. Before that I had had a fantastic body. I could wear anything. Now, even though I have lost the weight and regained my shape, I have these ugly stretch*

marks on my tummy that will never go away. It may sound silly, but I miss wearing that bikini!

What this woman really misses is the image she had of herself in that bikini—sexy, desirable. Her husband was probably quite attentive to her when she was dressed so flimsily. Husbands are the most often to blame in regard to their wives' feelings about their body image.

My husband looks at me and sighs, "You used to be so cute. But don't worry, you will soon be pretty and thin again." He says this as if he has underlined the word "thin." You can't be pretty unless you are thin too.

These accusations are largely cultural—being perpetrated by the notorious media. How can you compete with sixteen-year-old Brooke Shields? Having worked with models and done some modeling myself, I can say that modeling is chiefly a height and bone-structure issue. The rest of that beauty is taken care of by make-up, hair color, lighting, and the art of photo retouching. Unfortunately, we're led to believe that we should look like a photograph model, and when we stand in front of our unretouched mirrors, the results may be disappointing.

After you have had a baby, your body is not what you remembered it to be. Many women have weight to lose, and those that don't almost always have changed body proportions. Muscle groups lose tone and strength in pregnancy. The thighs, buttocks, breasts, abdomen, and upper arms tend to sag. It is not a comforting situation.

I feel like I am trapped in the wrong body. I know who I am or perhaps who I was, and it certainly isn't the person who accidentally "pees" in the kitchen while she's doing the dishes.

It may be that there are certain things you may not be able to change (stretch marks, for one thing, are often permanent). However, there are many that you can. But like any change, this demands commitment. The first step is to convince yourself that change is possible.

Many appearance flaws can be altered by the implementation of one or more of the following: 1) diet; 2) exercise; 3) posture; 4) cosmetic preparations. Once you look better physically, you will also begin to feel better about yourself.

The ultimate test I offer is to stand naked in front of a full-length mirror. This can be terrifying but it is also illuminating. Take a pad and pencil with you. Be resolved to stand in front of that mirror for a full five minutes without writing anything. This may be more difficult than you think. We often approach a mirror with the option of walking away. Take note of every part of your body—not just those that please or disgust you. Be objective. Look at your body as a whole, not just as a series of isolated parts. Now write down the feature that is the most outstanding in the positive sense. Is it your eyes, your hands, your legs? Now write down your weakest point. By this I mean the one feature that is most out of balance with the rest of you. Simply having "wide hips" is not negative, especially if you have a wide shoulder girdle and large breasts to match. Having "thin legs" may sound pleasing, but they may also be underdeveloped and need exercise to bring them to a more pleasing shape.

Now carefully analyze and write down specifically what you want to change. Put this paper away but remember to take it out at least once a day and look at it. There are some aspects that, though they cannot be changed in the literal sense, can be improved. Bone structure is one thing. Glandular structure is another. For instance, if you are 5'2½", you are never going to be 5'10". You can, however, appear taller by improving your posture and in some cases, through spinal exercise, increase your height by about one-half inch. The size of your breasts is also something that cannot be altered, without surgery. They can, however, be firm and well toned if you develop the pectoral muscle underneath the breast tissue.

Your muscle distribution is also something that is practically unchangeable. By this I do not mean fat. I'm talking about the structure and mass of your muscle tissue. If the muscles in either your arms or your legs are particularly large, it is extremely difficult to break them down and make them smaller. I would consider instead reshaping the muscle with proper exercise—lengthening and elongating these muscles so that they don't bunch together and appear lumpy.

Also, you must consider the concept of diet and exercise working together. Too many women substitute one for the other and wonder why they are not obtaining the desired results. Dieting alone isn't enough. You will just have a small, flabby body rather than a large, flabby one. Though exercise is essential, it alone cannot bring about significant weight loss. The information that follows, as well as the information included in Chapters Three and Four, will tell you specifically how to improve your physical self.

As a final note, remember a healthy body image can be gained only by seeing yourself as a total person. It doesn't really matter whether you are a size six or a size fourteen as long as you feel healthy and strong. Women come in all sizes and shapes. Your career, your family, your interests, and your body are part of you. Once you learn to integrate and balance both the physical and emotional aspects of your life, you will experience a kind of renaissance—a rebirth and a growing acceptance of yourself. And at the critical period after you have given birth, it's particularly helpful to achieve this.

"What Has Happened to My Body?" Your Postpartum Anatomy

Rather than present a cosmetic evaluation of your postpartum appearance here, I feel it more beneficial to discuss the physiology of the postpartum mother. There is a succession of natural events that follow delivery, and if they are unanticipated, they can cause unnecessary concern.

The physical changes of the body from full pregnancy through the first year

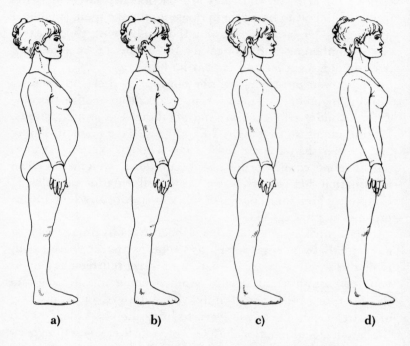

a)   b)   c)   d)

**a) Full pregnancy—8 months   b) Immediately after delivery
c) Six weeks after delivery   d) One year after delivery**

The first is the lochia. Lochia is a vaginal discharge, similar to that of menstruation, which occurs in the ten-to-twenty-day period following delivery. Technically the lochia is the remaining cells of the placental site and the uterine lining. It is quite red in color for the first few days and will be unusually heavy in comparison to your menstrual discharge. This reddish color fades on or about the tenth day to a yellowish-white color that is often blood-streaked. The last portion of the lochia is generally a white, mucous discharge. In most cases, due to the large amount of discharge, it is necessary to wear hospital-size sanitary napkins. These are larger than the standard sanitary napkin, almost the size of a disposable diaper. The peculiar odor of the lochia (some women have described it as smelling like a "rotten egg" or "spoiled milk") may be offensive to you, but usually can be remedied with proper hygiene, including the bathing and cleansing of the perineal area, which includes the clitoris, urethra, vagina, and anus; be clean and change the pad every two to three hours, and you should be fine.

Although vaginal hemorrhaging is not usual, it is still important to watch for it during this time (if hemorrhaging does occur, it normally happens during the twenty-day period in which the lochia is present). How do you know you are hemorrhaging? My midwife gave this rather graphic description. If your lochia spills out of your sanitary napkin and runs down the inside of your leg and into your shoe, you are hemorrhaging and you had better go to the hospital. Severe hemorrhaging is fairly uncommon. If your lochia continues for more than four weeks or if the bright red bleeding continues for more than two weeks, consult your doctor.

Many obstetricians administer an episiotomy before the actual delivery. This procedure involves the cutting of the vaginal lips to prevent the tissues being torn. This severance is stitched after the baby has been delivered. If you have had an episiotomy, keep the stitches moist. Vitamin A&D or vitamin E creams are excellent moisturizers. If the stitches dry out, they have a tendency to pull and can cause unnecessary pain and discomfort. If your stitches are still irritating after moisturizing, your physician can recommend specific treatments. In general, the pain of episiotomy repair is caused simply by edema or the accumulation of vaginal fluids in the stitches. If you keep this area clean, you can avoid most problems. Until your stitches are completely healed, the use of tampons or douching is generally not recommended.

For a day or two, and sometimes longer after delivery, you may experience constipation or incontinence, the inability to control urination.

You may urinate involuntarily, especially when coughing or laughing. If necessary, constipation can be remedied with a gentle laxative. More than likely, you will move your bowels within seventy-two hours of delivery. Constipation is generally caused by fatigued pelvic muscles, weakened by delivery, and it can be treated with proper pelvic exercise, which I describe in Chapter Three.

If it is impossible for you to urinate due to a prolonged or a forceps or a breech delivery—which can weaken your bladder muscles—you may need to have a tube passed into your bladder to facilitate elimination. This process is known as catheterization and is a quite painless procedure.

Even when you return home, your bladder and bowel movements will not be normal. Highly aerobic or strenuous exercise during the two weeks after delivery is not recommended, due to your weakened pelvic muscles. However, the essential pelvic exercises I recommend later on, if practiced with the permission of your physician, are encouraged, to relieve your bladder and bowel symptoms.

The puerperium is the time when the uterus and other genital organs return to their normal size. This process is also referred to as "involution." After delivery, the uterus weighs about two and a half pounds; after two weeks it weighs eleven ounces; and finally, after six to eight weeks, it returns to its prepregnant weight of two ounces.

The cervix, vagina, and external genitalia—which have been stretched to capacity during delivery—gradually regain their muscle tone over an eight-week period. The degree of muscle tone regained is largely dependent on your conscientious exercise efforts during pregnancy. If you have not exercised, your muscles will remain slack and will need to be re-toned with postpartum exercise (see Chapter Three).

For the first few days after birth, your breasts will produce a clear, bluish fluid known as colostrum (see Chapter Four, on breast-feeding). You may have noticed this excretion also during your pregnancy. This thin fluid, though not milk in the real sense, contains substances extremely valuable to your baby. These substances are nature's antibodies, which protect your newborn from disease during these early days. Your breasts and nipples may become engorged and painful, and the areola, the circular area surrounding the nipples, will darken in color. If your breasts do become engorged and you do not choose to breast-feed your baby, you may apply ice packs to your breasts and restrict your fluid intake for several days to relieve this discomfort. Nursing mothers can learn to express their milk either manually or with a breast pump, which I will discuss in Chapter Four. Mothers not breast-feeding their babies can also express their milk to relieve engorgement, but expression encourages increased milk production, and this is not generally recommended unless the mother intends to nurse the baby. Your physician will be able to prescribe treatments for you if your nipples become inflamed or irritated.

It is particularly at this point, when your body begins to produce milk, that many mothers may experience their most extreme depression. This extreme reaction is largely due to hormonal changes. Your level of estrogen, which is essential to the growth of your uterine lining and to the development of your mammary duct tissue, drops drastically after delivery. However, progesterone (the hormone responsible for thickening the uterine lining so that conception can occur), prolactin, and PHT, the hormones responsible for lactation, continue to be produced by your postpartum system in relatively large amounts, to ensure adequate milk production. The juxtapositioning of these hormone levels causes a temporary yet sudden endocrine imbalance similar to your premenstrual state. The January 1978 issue of the journal *Psychoneuroendocrinology*[1] states that the correlation between prolactin and PRL (another hormone involved in the lactation process) in conjunction with estrogen and the low progesterone levels following delivery, may be responsible for depressive symptoms such as anxiety and irritability. The doctors involved in this study sometimes prescribed artificial progesterone injections to relieve some of the symptoms of postpartum depression. However, according to the journal *Medical Hypotheses*,[2] the etiology of these hormonal imbalances is still rather vague. Though these experts believe that both endorphins* and estrogen are involved in postpartum depression, there is no firm documentation of their exact function.

These previously described hormones, so necessary to adequate milk production, do possess some less-than-desirable properties. They keep your muscles softer and ensure a larger proportion of fatty tissue production than there would be if you chose not to breast-feed your baby, since a fat surplus in the body is necessary for adequate milk production. The milk-producing hormones also contribute to a general fatigue and lethargy. These properties should not discourage you from breast-feeding your child. It is still the safest and most nutritious method of feeding your baby. Also, the hormones released during lactation help shrink your uterus back to its prepregnant state more quickly than if you chose not to nurse the baby. This is why, while you are breast-feeding him, you may experience milk contractions in your uterus. These contractions should not upset you but rather delight you, as they are indicating the shrinking of your uterus back to its normal size. The uterus of a mother not breast-feeding her child will also shrink, but not quite so quickly.

Your body, though it may be slim, will be softer and less strong due to the lactation hormones. Your abdomen, buttocks, and thighs will be particularly loose and flabby during this time. Proper exercise can accelerate the restoration of your former muscle tone, so exercise as soon as your doctor allows. Even if you choose not to breast-feed your baby, you may still experience lethargy and depression, due to factors such as fa-

* Endorphins are the amino acids (protein) found in the brain that control a number of physiological responses including the suppression of pain.

tigue and lack of exercise. It has also been theorized that there are unknown hormones present in the postpartum mother that are uninvolved in lactation, and these hormones may also be responsible for feelings of depression. It is known, however, that your body takes a full twelve months to return completely to its prepregnant state both structurally and hormonally.

A similar hormonal imbalance is evident prior to menstruation, so if you are generally irritable and depressed prior to your period, you may feel the same way during your postpartum recovery. Your postpartum depression, however, will be more dramatic than your premenstrual condition because of the greater intensity of hormonal fluctuations after pregnancy.

If you have a cesarean section (the delivery of the baby surgically through the abdomen rather than vaginally), you may have to wait a longer time before you can resume abdominal exercise. Your abdominal muscles have been severed during surgery and will need time to heal. There is usually no need to worry about cesarean scars today. The "bikini line" incision that is the preferred cesarean technique is barely noticeable. You will also need greater perseverance in your abdominal exercises than a woman who has delivered vaginally. Your weakened abdominal muscles will need greater attention, to restore firm, flat abdominal support.

About six weeks after delivery, you should have a postnatal examination. During this exam, your doctor will check your uterus to make certain it has resumed its normal size. He will question you about abdominal pain and vaginal discharges. A blood test may be given, to check for anemia. Your weight and blood pressure will be measured, and your breasts will be checked; also, if you have had an episiotomy, the stitches will be checked to make certain they have healed. The doctor will also check for any inflammation or erosion of the cervix. Twenty-five percent of all first pregnancies have some degree of cervical erosion. Cervical erosion is a disorder of the uterus which occurs when the cells lining the cervical canal extend down until they are visible at the mouth of the vagina. There is no need for treatment unless this condition lasts for longer than six months or is accompanied by vaginal discharge.

Most physicians favor the delaying of sexual intercourse until you have had your postpartum exam. If, however, you did not undergo an episiotomy and you are otherwise healthy, and your lochia has ceased, you may with your doctor's consent resume sexual activity before this time. If intercourse is painful, try taking a hot bath and lubricating your vagina with vitamin E cream. If you still experience pain or muscular cramps during intercourse, consult your doctor.

Unfortunately, if you have stretch marks on your stomach or legs, there is little you can do about them. The secret to avoiding stretch marks is in prevention, not in cure. It's a good idea to smooth on vitamin E oil or a similar preparation over your breasts, abdomen, buttocks, and thighs during pregnancy itself. The elasticity this moisturizing ensures can help in keeping your skin smooth and free of marks. The linea negra, or "black line," which appears between your navel and genitalia during your pregnancy, is in a sense also a stretch mark. It is, however, unavoidable: it represents the division of your stomach muscles, to accommodate the fetus. The darkened pigmentation of the linea negra, produced by hormones secreted in pregnancy, does fade in the postpartum period but will always be slightly evident to the trained eye. If you have not taken sufficient precautions to avoid stretch marks during pregnancy, the best you can hope for is to fade these stretch marks gradually, but they will never disappear. The best preparations for fading your stretch marks consist of vitamins A, D, and E, and cocoa butter. These can be purchased in almost any pharmacy, or in a cosmetic or health-food store. Some of these preparations are messy, even waxy in consistency, but they are the only ointments that produce the desired effect. Just baby oil or petroleum jelly is not enough. If you are nursing your child, be sure to apply generous amounts of lubricants to your breasts. The continual enlargement and deflation of your breasts due to nursing can contribute to new or further stretch marks. If you do use these preparations on your breasts, be sure to clean your areolae and nipples before feeding your infant. These preparations may contain chemicals that are best not ingested by your baby.

Your menstruation normally returns within twenty-four weeks if you are breast-feeding your child and within six to ten weeks if you are not. The first menstruation is almost always unusual in some way. There may be clots, or it may be unusually heavy. It may stop and then start again. Your second period is likely to be close to normal. If you breast-feed the baby, you will ovulate after the twentieth week. This delay of ovulation has caused some women to view nursing as a form of contraception. Though you are less likely to conceive than someone who chooses to bottle-feed a child, you are not immune to pregnancy. I have known several women who have had to proceed with an involuntary weaning at their baby's six-month birthday because they had not undertaken a more reliable form of birth control and thus had become pregnant. If you do become pregnant, physicians suggest that you wean your nursing child gradually but do not continue to breast-feed him during your pregnancy, since your body and the new fetus require the best nourishment possible during gestation.

More than 10 percent of all pregnant women get varicose veins before the birth of their first child. Varicosities in the legs are caused by defective valves in the pelvis and are aggravated by the pressure of your enlarged uterus on the veins of your abdomen. Modern science has demonstrated that a varicose vein is formed when a clot blocks the passage of blood through a vein, causing it to become inflamed and irritated. Sometimes the vein becomes so severely clogged that no blood passage is possible.

In experiments as early as 1931, scientists proved that the lack of vitamin E in the bloodstream can cause varicosities during pregnancy. Generally, pregnant women who have developed varicose veins have had extremely limited amounts of vitamin E in their systems. The reason that lack of vitamin E in the bloodstream can contribute to varicosities is the following. Clots that normally form in the veins are composed of dead blood tissue. Since vitamin E aids in the development of new blood cells, to help replace the dead cells that form into clots, if there isn't any vitamin E available, the clot composed of dead tissue remains and grows larger. It is sad to think how many women suffer needlessly with this condition, which gradually grows worse with each subsequent pregnancy. Adequate amounts of vitamin E (do consult with a nutritionally informed physician for exact dosage information) have now proved to relieve greatly or even entirely eliminate varicosities without the traditional surgery. Some physicians may disagree with vitamin therapy techniques as a cure for varicose veins and will still recommend, instead, the use of elastic stockings to relieve the pain of varicosities. In my opinion, however, this view is extremely limited. There are many nutritionally minded physicians who advocate the use of vitamin therapies for such conditions as varicose veins. *Note:* Women with high blood pressure should use caution in taking vitamin E, since vitamin E has a tendency to raise the blood pressure in people who are not accustomed to it. Women with high blood pressure can still take small doses of vitamin E if they are under a doctor's supervision.

There are several conditions resulting from pregnancy which are overlooked because they do not occur in all postpartum mothers. They are, however, common enough to be included in a discussion of postpartum recovery. The first is prolapse, or the downward deplacement of the uterus. In prolapse the pelvic muscles, weakened by the strain of labor and delivery, are no longer able to support the uterus. The uterus sinks down into the vagina. The symptoms of prolapse include frequent and difficult urination, vaginal discharge, and lower back pain. Mild prolapses generally do not require treatment, except for prescribed pelvic exercise. Ninety-nine percent of all prolapses are the result of childbirth, although any heavy physical activity may contribute to this condition. More severe cases may require some form of surgery or the insertion of a pessary, a vaginal device placed at the neck of the womb to support the uterus.

The second is cuts and abrasions incurred by the baby's passage through the birth canal, which can cause vaginal infections. Though vaginal discharges are normal and expected during the postpartum period, chafing, itching, or burning of the vagina, vulva, or thighs should be discussed with your doctor, who will be best able to advise you on the proper treatment for these irritations.

The third condition, inflammation of the urethra (urethritis) or of the bladder (cystitis), is also common after childbirth. Tissue damage during delivery is often the cause. The symptoms include frequent urination—sometimes as often as every two to three minutes, pain during urination, and a feeling of extreme urgency to urinate even when there is no urine to pass. This again is something to discuss with your doctor. Chronic urethritis or cystitis can be serious, and can be eradicated only through the careful guidance of your physician.

In conclusion, I would like to reiterate that most physiological results of childbirth, like the corresponding emotional responses, are perfectly normal. They may seem to be extraordinary at the time, but keep in mind that they are common, and with proper nutrition, exercise, and psychological support you can overcome them. The key to coping actively with the physiological changes which occur during the postpartum period lies in first educating yourself as fully as possible about these physiological changes; second, in maintaining a close relationship with your gynecologist, and third, by being patient with yourself. These physiological changes are not permanent. They will disappear with perseverance and the guidance of your physician.

THE FACTS ABOUT FAT

The best protection against becoming fat during pregnancy and the postpartum period is never to become fat. Most of us are the victims of the junk-food era. We grew up with a chocolate bar in one hand and a Twinkie in the other. We sacrificed nutrition for "goodies." We were rewarded with cookies and fattening desserts.

All I ever remember about childhood is desserts. The Good Humor man was a deity in our neighborhood. I choked down my dinner to get to the "good stuff" faster.

As puberty approached, some of us took a look at our pudgy little bodies, became frustrated, and, prompted by peer pressure, went on whatever fad diet was popular at that time. A typical fad-diet strategy would be to eat nothing but hard-boiled eggs and tomatoes for two to three days. Then, when we broke down from mental hunger and malnutrition, we would open a box of chocolate doughnuts or some other fattening food and devour it all.

We would repeat this cycle again the next week—starting with a new diet, which recommended your eating nothing but bananas for two to three days. This kind of physical abuse had nothing but disastrous effects. Our body weight went totally out of control—going up and down from binge to diet, from binge to diet. The fashion magazines added to our neurosis by presenting pages and pages of undernourished models wearing miniskirts, whom we strove to duplicate.

It is a known fact that eating disturbances and depression tend to coincide. American women have the highest rate of eating disorders (see Chapter One) of any single group. And it is therefore not surprising that they also have the highest rate of depression.

The erratic eating patterns of adolescence tend to follow us into adulthood. Never is this more evident than with the onset of pregnancy. Thirty years ago, doctors prescribed strict diets in which the pregnant mother was carefully monitored, and was humiliated if she gained more than fifteen pounds; that level of strictness, I feel, is too severe. This practice led to a vast increase in premature babies. Today's obstetrician maintains a more conservative view concerning weight gain. Twenty-five pounds is now the normal expectation. Statistics show that the average American woman gains twenty-nine pounds during her pregnancy; this means that almost 50 percent of these women gain more than is recommended.

It is not the actual weight gain that is so disturbing; it is the way in which women gain that weight. Our great-grandmothers often gained thirty to forty pounds during their pregnancies, yet were able to lose this weight easily. But this was in the days of unprocessed foods—such as fresh fruits and vegetables, whole grains, and homemade dairy products—and of hard physical labor. What they did not lose in delivery they lost in sweat, plowing the ground or doing housework. If they had a bit of fat left on them they were often grateful.

Today 20 percent of all women begin their pregnancy overweight. Add to this an additional twenty-nine pounds gathered, and you may have a woman who has to lose fifty or sixty pounds during the postpartum period to return to a desirable weight. Overweight people are not healthy people. The woman who looks like a seventeenth-century Rubens nude, with her ample posterior—who is often cited as the zenith in "big beauties"—is not a healthy woman. She is old at thirty and suffers all the ailments commonly associated with obesity, including lower-back pain, hypertension, and diabetes. She is not only physically but mentally lethargic. She is short of breath, her joints ache, and she has poor digestion. She has difficult pregnancies and subsequent deliveries. She is more likely to have high blood pressure, heart disease, kidney disorders, cirrhosis of the liver, pneumonia, inflammation of the gall bladder, arthritis, and varicose veins than her slimmer counterparts.

In some cases, the more lenient attitude on the part of doctors has caused today's woman to view pregnancy as a nine-month binge. The attitude is "Well, if I am going to gain weight anyway, why not have a good time?" But Coca-Cola and chocolate cake do not a healthy mommy or a healthy baby make. Still, many women use their pregnancies as a time for unhealthful overindulgence. Perhaps it is the only time they have had an excuse to be fat. In other words, there are thousands of good excuses to be overweight but no good reasons.

On the other side of the coin, there is the healthy, sensible woman, who has monitored her eating habits, not indulging in crash diets or binges; who exercises religiously; who during her pregnancy may even gain the same twenty-nine pounds by eating healthy, nutritious food; and who six weeks after delivery is showing off the same shape she had previous to her pregnancy.

So it is not how much you eat, but what you eat and the way you eat that is important. This is not an excuse to go out and gain forty pounds when your doctor tells you to gain twenty-five, but it is a plug for the quality of food and the maintenance of sound eating habits.

This may be as good a time as any to take a look at the methods by which our bodies process food and some of the reasons women become overweight. Food, in a sense, is a form of chemical energy. Living things need sources of energy simply to continue such life functions as growth, repair, and motion. The basic unit for measuring energy is the scientist's calorie. Your calorie needs are measured in direct proportion to your height, your age, and the amount of physical activity you engage in. The average woman may utilize between 1200 and 1800 calories in a normal day. If you are pregnant, you should increase your caloric intake by about 300 calories, and if you are breast-feeding your baby, you should increase it by 500 calories. If, through your life processes or physical activity, you fail to use all of the calories you have ingested in the form of food energy, your body will develop fat deposits. Thin people also store fat in their bodies, but the overweight person's fat storage far exceeds any normal future demand.

The structure of particular food cells can also determine whether or not a specific person can become overweight. Let's use my previous example of two pregnant women—the one who gains the average twenty-nine pounds during her pregnancy by eating wholesome foods and the other, gaining the same amount of weight by eating "junk" food. Why can the woman who eats wholesome foods lose her excess postpartum weight more quickly than the woman who has eaten the "junk" food? The reason is this. Food which we have come to label as "junk" is largely the lower carbohydrates—sugar and starch. The body has a difficult time assimilating these substances because there are so few nutrients to be broken down in these foods. Whole foods, on the other hand, and the nutrients they contain, are easily absorbed by the body and changed into energy that can be utilized. The "junk" food is simply turned into fat, because nutrients are not present in these foods.

"But I have always been overweight," you complain, and "I hardly eat a thing." I am always wary of the person who uses these defenses. No one is naturally fat. Many people have so many unconscious eating habits firmly meshed in their lives that they don't even know when and what they are eating. They munch in front of the TV or while reading. They order a diet plate at lunch and proceed to nibble off everyone else's plate. Cheating serves no one, least of all yourself. "I have big bones" or "It's my glands"—these are two other common defenses. Variations in bone density can rarely account for more than a seven-pound weight difference, and only a fraction of a percent of overweight people can attribute their problem to hormonal disturbances.

The first question you must ask yourself is "Do I really want to lose weight?" If your answer is yes, then ask yourself why. If you want to lose weight for anyone else, other than yourself—think again. Your weight loss must be your own reward, not someone else's.

Now I'd like to address a special group of women, whom I'll call the "chronic dieters." You are basically healthy but you want to be ten pounds lighter. To be ten pounds lighter, you diet severely and in an essentially un-nutritious manner. When you begin to eat in your normal, nutritious way again, the ten pounds come crawling back. Your scale has been like a seesaw—up and down, up and down. Medical professionals now feel that this constant gaining and losing of weight is actually more hazardous than keeping that ten pounds on. I agree; health is the most important thing, not just merely being "thin." Exercise may be what you need. And if you tighten your muscles, your body will actually appear thinner.

The culprit of most overweight problems is bad eating habits. You always hear ". . . but my whole family is fat." True, your family may well be fat, but the fat is not in their genes. It is in their habits. If you are a mother breast-feeding a baby, you have reason to be an additional three to five pounds over your normal weight, due to retained fluids and breast weight. But if you weigh more than that, it is time for a little self-examination. The results of bad eating habits often surface during periods of stress. Adolescence, pregnancy, the postpartum period, and menopause are the four most likely times for a woman to gain excess weight. They also represent the greatest periods of emotional strain in a woman's life. Hormones are partially responsible for this, but heavily ingrained habits are more often the cause. We live in a society obsessed with food. Advertisements constantly offer to sell us something new to eat. It is ironic to note that the two most popular kinds of books year after year are cookbooks and diet books; are we not supposed to eat what we have just cooked?

An essential factor in evaluating your eating habits is to ask yourself if you are really hungry. If you really want to lose weight, you have to be able to answer that question. The truth is that most of us don't know the answer. We eat automatically—perhaps because it is lunchtime or because we are going to a party. The normally effective appetite control mechanism in our brains gets confused. It keeps sending down messages, but we keep ignoring them. Pretty soon, we get confused too and aren't really sure we are truly hungry.

The first rule of any effective weight loss and maintenance program is to eat only when you are hungry. Thin people do this naturally. They may skip a meal here and there but never in the name of dieting. They simply are not hungry. Skinny people also eat rich, fattening desserts, but when they are full they leave that last bit of ice cream in the bowl. They've had their fill. When they are really hungry for ice cream again, they know they can have some because they only eat what their body needs and no more. The overweight person eats the same ice cream, feels guilty, and has a second or a third bowl to mask his or her feelings. There are many excuses to eat more than your body needs. What I am trying to point out is that the thin person and the overweight person can eat the very same foods. The difference in their consumption is in their attitudes and in the habits they have formed about food. Most of the time, the thin person eats only because he or she is hungry. The overweight person is often eating for a variety of other reasons. Most of the time when the overweight person eats, he or she is not hungry at all.

It is difficult to be able to identify true hunger after years of eating "under false pretenses," but it can be done. The symptoms of true hunger are fairly conspicuous. When your body needs food, the appetite control mechanism sends a little message down to your stomach and then back to your brain. Your body responds with a mild contracting sensation in your stomach. I am not talking about excruciating pain. If you get headaches or become dizzy from dieting, then you are going too long without food. Your stomach may growl, or you may even get cramps if you are famished.

On the other hand, when you do become hungry, by all means eat, but eat only what you need. We all know the story of the conscientious dieters who starve themselves throughout the day and devour everything in sight that evening. They actually consume more in a single hour than they would if they ate sparingly throughout the day. That is why I favor the concept of "minimeals"—eating several small meals per day rather than two or three large ones. Though it is still the subject of controversy, there is evidence that some people burn up their surplus fat in a process called thermogenesis. After every meal, there is a rise in the body's metabolic rate. Though two people may actually eat exactly the same amount of exactly the same foods, the person who has eaten the smaller, more frequent, meals will burn up more calories than the person who has eaten two or three large meals.

Eating small amounts of food when you are hungry also abates your appetite. Snacking between meals has always been a "no-no." "Don't eat that. It will spoil your appetite" was the warning. What does that matter? So you will have one serving of potatoes instead of three or maybe you won't have any. Isn't that what you want to do—curb your eating? Of course, it can depend on what kind of snack you choose. An apple, a slice of cheese, a half cup of yogurt, or even an oatmeal cookie can be filling and nutritious. Later on, at dinner, leave something on your plate or take a little less. By eating less, you will soon find you won't be hungry enough to finish everything.

I found these "minimeals" especially necessary during the postpartum period. The new hormones in your body are making you tired as it is. As the eating of heavy meals tends to make you sleepy, smaller, evenly spaced, more frequent meals will give you energy without creating lethargy. If you are breast-feeding your baby, it also helps you to adapt to his schedule. You eat a little, and then so does your baby. It works very well. When you are eating small amounts of food regularly, that overfull feeling from fewer but larger meals will make you uncomfortable. Stomach sizes are essentially the same, regardless of your height and weight. They are roughly the size of a loose fist and can hold at maximum about two and a fourth pints of food. When you are overweight, you grow accustomed to stretching your stomach beyond its limit. This "stuffed" feeling, which would make a person of normal weight uncomfortable, is not perceivable when you're used to stretching your stomach, and so you continue to eat. However, when your food has been digested, your stomach returns to the same size as anyone else's.

The next concept I feel necessary to successful weight loss

is the idea of being "fussy." You remember your mother telling you, "Don't pick at your food. Don't be so fussy." If you are overweight you will probably say that you will eat almost anything. Maybe you can, but do you like almost anything? I will, of course, discuss foods in more detail in the next section, but the fact is that there are some foods we like and some foods we simply do not. Our bodies require a certain amount of nutrition, so we should choose our foods from a nutritional point of view, not simply for pleasure. There are some foods which are positively unpalatable, yet we should include them in our diets to ensure good health. The point is that there is no person who enjoys absolutely all foods. But how many times do we eat something simply because it is there? We may sample a certain food that is not particularly nutritionally beneficial, that we do not really enjoy but we still continue to eat it. We look into the refrigerator, find nothing appetizing there, and yet still have something to eat. How many times have you seen the dessert tray in a restaurant and, though none of your favorites were there, have still taken something?

Often when you are in the mood for a particular food, it is only that food which will remove your hunger. If you can afford it, include certain nutritious treats in your food shopping to satisfy cravings in a healthful way. If you enjoy shrimp, figs, or pumpernickel, buy them. Why suffer with eggs and grapefruit if you don't really like them? If you are going to eat several enjoyable and nutritious and yet collectively low-caloric foods during the day, you will not be starving from either physical or mental hunger.

You must learn to change your thinking about so-called "fattening" foods. No one food is inherently fattening or inherently dietetic. Try to consider whether a food is inherently nutritious instead. Again, your choice of food must depend on the amount of it you consume and on what particular food is going to satisfy your hunger. Three ounces of lean hamburger, one slice of custard pie, one medium sweet potato, two slices of American cheese, or three cups of Brussels sprouts all have about 200 calories. You may not want to eat all of those Brussels sprouts, even though you've been told that the cheese and those other suggestions are not on your diet plan. Those two slices of cheese, however, may satisfy your hunger. All of those Brussels sprouts will only make you sick if you don't like them, and you still may be hungry after eating them because they aren't satisfying you. Be selective about the foods you eat. What good are all of these "diet foods" if you can't bear to eat them?

If you adhere to all of the formerly mentioned eating suggestions—1) to eat only when you are truly hungry; 2) to stop eating when you are full (leave something on your plate); and 3) to be selective about the foods you eat—then you have mastered the three basic weight-control statutes. You will be well on your way to a lifetime of "thin thinking" about food.

"AM I EATING THE RIGHT THINGS?" YOUR NUTRITIONAL NEEDS

The answer to this question, as far as postpartum recovery is concerned, is largely determined by your decision about whether or not to breast-feed your child. If you do choose to (see Chapter Four), your nutritional requirements will be of greater consequence than when you were pregnant. I am not referring just to the intake of calories. Merely consuming an additional 500 to 800 calories per day is not going to furnish you with a healthy milk supply. What is really important is food value. Whether or not you are trying to lose weight, your body requires a minimum of nutrients to function properly. When you are breast-feeding a child, your need for these nutrients increases significantly. You are no longer responsible merely for your nutrition and that of a seven-to-eight pound fetus but for the completely separate life functions of your infant, who could weigh fifteen to eighteen pounds in less than a year's time. If your body does not receive these nutrients, not only will you be unable to maintain a weight loss effectively but you will be exposing both you and your infant to a variety of infections.

If you do nothing else for yourself, limit your intake of white, processed sugar. The average American woman eats 125 pounds of processed sugar each year. I am not just concerned that sugar and the foods which are processed with it are high in calories, which, of course, they are, but that they are potentially detrimental to your physical well-being. You can have an occasional dish of ice cream or a slice of cake without risking weight gain, but most American women eat sugar daily and in relatively large amounts—about a third of a pound of sugar per day. This outlandish consumption is not exclusively your fault. Sugar is hidden in many foods. Seemingly innocent foods such as canned soup, ketchup, bread, and luncheon meats are processed with varying amounts of sugar. You must learn either to read labels or to prepare these foods yourself.

Why is sugar so bad? There are several reasons. For one thing, it causes tooth decay. Sugary fluids accumulate on your gums and teeth, promoting an acid medium for bacteria to grow in. If you breast-feed your baby, the sugar you take into your body goes directly into your breast milk, predisposing your infant to tooth and gum infections. Since white sugar is so highly processed, it has lost any nutritive value it might have once possessed as a sugar beet. Processed sugar is more like a drug than a food, because, like a drug, it stimulates the body without nourishing it. We get an immediate "high" from sugar, as we would from any stimulant, and then that "high" quickly subsides into fatigue. In order for sugar to be absorbed in the body, considerable quantities of such vitamins and minerals as thiamine, riboflavin, niacin, pyridoxine, pantothenic acid, phosphorus, and magnesium must be used. Thus, if a mother and her breast-fed infant regularly ingest sugar and do not adequately replenish these nutrients, they are bound to end up with some vitamin and mineral deficiencies. Sugar can also promote diabetes, hypoglycemia, and diarrhea. It can also produce surprising changes in disposition. Breast-fed infants who are given sugar tend to be irritable and cranky. They also develop a taste for sweets that may cause problems in their adult lives.

Learn to use sugar substitutes (but not saccharin!). Honey, date sugar, natural maple syrup, molasses, and fresh fruit are all whole foods. They, unlike processed sugars, can be broken down and metabolized by the body like any other balanced carbohydrate.

Americans consume about fifteen pounds of salt annually, and this amount is substantially over any normal requirement. This is not to say that salt should be avoided completely, but it should be taken in moderation. Sea salt, kelp, and other natural salts are beneficial to both mother and baby, as they provide the vital nutrient iodine in substantial quantities. If you suffer from high blood pressure or water retention, then, of course, yours is a different situation. Your physician can advise on salt restrictions in these cases. Salt can, if ingested above the required amounts, cause digestive disturbances in breast-fed infants. If you notice your baby frequently spitting up food, or being generally uncomfortable and crying during feeding, salt reduction may be the answer. Again, always consult your pediatrician if anything unusual occurs.

White, enriched flour is also something to be wary of whether or not you choose to breast-feed your baby. In our grandmothers' day, bread was the "staff of life." It contained rich whole grains, whole eggs, and fresh butter. It was a completely balanced food, containing protein, carbohydrates, and fat. Today most of these valuable nutrients have been flushed away by modern technology. A slice of white bread has very little nutritional value. And don't allow the word "enriched" to deceive you. All this means is that after the manufacturer has pulverized all of the twenty-odd nutrients out of that stalk of wheat, he has had the decency to put four of them back. Whole grains are one of the most valuable foods a new mother can eat. Don't cheat yourself. Wheat germ, oatmeal, and brown rice are bursting with nutrients. If you can find the time to bake, use whole-grain flours.

The food value of caffeine is fairly negligible. Though it has been used effectively to treat some disorders, such as migraine headaches and low blood pressure, in most instances it tends to disturb the system. Coffee and tea, like processed sugar, are drugs. They stimulate the body for a time, while they draw valuable nutrients out of your body. If you tend to be stimulated by these beverages, your breast-fed infant will be likewise. The best thing to do, if you feel that you must have an occasional cup, is to drink it with meals. The mixture of food with caffeine tends to lessen its stimulating properties.

Though you have been encouraged to avoid alcohol for the duration of your pregnancy, both your obstetrician and your pediatrician may suggest a glass of wine or beer in the evening if you are breast-feeding your child. Alcohol is a depressant and will help you relax. If you are relaxed, your milk will flow more easily. Beer is also rich in yeast, a nutrient vital to the production of high-quality breast milk.

Protein is the basis of any living organism. It is the only food constituent that contains nitrogen—an element necessary to maintain the chemical balance in the brain, the spine, and the intestines. Severe deficiencies of this nutrient can cause anemia, kidney disease, poor circulation, and weak muscle tone. People who go without protein foods for prolonged periods can expect to age rapidly, the body becoming flabby and the facial muscles losing tone and becoming wrinkled. Proteins consist of about twenty-two complex substances known as amino acids. These amino acids can be found in both animals and plants. Because animal proteins contain all of the essential amino acids, they are considered complete proteins. Plant proteins, in most cases, contain fewer of these amino acids and thus must be combined with each other to form complete proteins. Vegetarians can, if they combine their foods effectively, receive adequate protein for breast-feeding. If you are a lacto-ovo vegetarian—a vegetarian who eats dairy foods and eggs (as opposed to a true vegetarian, who eats only foods from plant sources), you are better off, for you will be able to receive your amino-acid requirements also from several complete proteins.

How many grams of protein do you need daily? The recommendation is about one gram for every 2.2 pounds of body weight. If you divide your desirable weight in half you should arrive at the correct amount. For instance, if you weigh or want to weigh 110 pounds, you should eat 55 grams of protein daily. If you are breast-feeding a baby, add an additional 20 grams. This is as simple as adding a couple of eggs or three ounces of tuna to your meal plan.

Of course, protein recommendations for mothers breast-feeding their babies continue to vary. The British medical association believes you should eat 100 grams. In Ghana, a mother breast-feeding a child eats only about 40 grams of protein, with only one quarter of that derived from animal sources, yet she is able to nurse her child until he is four to five years old. She may even nurse several children at the same time. To eat more than the recommended protein allowance may be all right, but one point has to be taken into consideration—protein cannot be stored in the body for very long, so whatever you don't use is essentially wasted. However, the lack of adequate protein can be more serious. It can result in fatigue, constipation, poor vision, and nervous instability.

The best sources of vegetable protein are legumes, seeds, sprouts, and nuts. The soybean is the most complete of vegetable proteins, followed closely by brewer's yeast. Many of you may gag just thinking about these foods. It's true, they are none too appetizing for many. However, the fact remains that one cup of low-fat soy flour has a full 60 grams of protein, and one-half cup of brewer's yeast has about 20 grams. You can purchase a concentrated soy flour combined with brewer's yeast. There are many such products on the market, some laced with fructose sweetener (fruit sugar) to make them more palatable. When you get up in the morning, place two tablespoons of this preparation in your blender with one-half cup of orange or apple juice or one-half cup of milk, and blend. This instant breakfast food is loaded with protein and other nutrients and is completely balanced because it contains both animal (if you use milk) and vegetable proteins. It is a quick, easy, and light meal, which makes it so desirable for postpartum mothers. You may even grow to enjoy it. It has about 110 calories and can count as one of your minimeals.

This kind of morning "toddy," when prepared with juice, is especially good if you are allergic to milk and milk products, as I am. It helps to replenish your milk supply without your resorting to dairy products.

Though I am strongly in favor of the inclusion of animal proteins in the postpartum diet, I still expect you to be selective about the animal proteins you choose. Many farm animals have been injected with antibiotics and hormones that are not necessarily hygienic or beneficial. It is true that you can find something wrong with almost anything you eat, but fish from deep sea levels—such as swordfish, blackfish, and tile fish with low mercury levels—eggs, yogurt, and cheese seem to be more free of pollutants than other animal products. As we grow older, our ability to digest milk and milk products decreases; the enzymes that help to absorb lactose are available only in extremely minute amounts. Thus when you buy cheese, it is important to look for the word "enzymes" in the list of ingredients. If you are not buying prepackaged cheese, ask your grocer to show you the ingredients listed on his wholesale products. This way you will know that the food you are buying can be metabolized by you and your baby. Otherwise, cheese becomes virtually a "dead food," unable to give adequate nutrition.

Next on our list of foods is carbohydrates. Carbohydrates have been given a bad name in recent years. They have been accused of causing obesity and high blood pressure. The carbohydrates are not, however, at fault in and of themselves. It is the *kind* of carbohydrates we Americans insist on eating that is to blame. Doughnuts, macaroni, and white rice are all highly processed foods with empty calories. Natural whole carbohydrates, however, play a vital role in the proper functioning of our internal organs and of our central nervous system, and in heart and muscle contraction. Fresh, raw fruit and vegetables provide adequate amounts of carbohydrates.

Fats are our most concentrated form of food energy. While one ounce of protein or carbohydrates produces about 113 calories in the human body, the same amount of fat produces 225 calories. Fat provides insulation and protection for body structures and internal organs. There are two basic types of fat—saturated and unsaturated. Both of these types of fat melt when heated and harden when cooled. Saturated fat, however, hardens at room temperature and if consumed regularly can result in high blood-cholesterol levels. These cholesterol levels can produce certain types of heart disease. This, however, does not mean that you should not eat fats. On the contrary, unsaturated fats, as found in liquid vegetable oils, are extremely vital to the functioning of your sex glands and the assimilation of fat-soluble vitamins. Fat-free diets, once thought to be beneficial, are now being discovered as unhealthful and even hazardous. One nutrition journal reports that there is actually more weight loss on a high-fat diet than on a high-carbohydrate diet. Fat abates your appetite and actually helps you to burn excess fat. The best unsaturated fats to include in your diet are safflower, corn, cod-liver, sunflower, sesame, and soybean oils.

Water, though not a nutrient in the true sense, makes up about two-thirds of our bodies. Its function is to transport foods to the appropriate tissues and to carry away the waste products to be excreted. The average daily requirement is about six to eight glasses of water per day. Some of this water already exists in food, so it is not always necessary to drink six to eight glasses to get the required amount of liquid.

Vitamins are chemical substances found in the foods we eat. The body does not manufacture these substances, so it is essential that we choose our vitamin-rich foods carefully. Vitamins do not provide heat or energy in the body the way that proteins or carbohydrates do, but they do perform the vital role of regulating chemical processes in the body and protecting the body against disease and illness. There are forty known vitamin substances, and twelve of these have proved themselves intrinsic to proper growth and development. There are basically two types of vitamins—fat-soluble and water-soluble. Fat-soluble vitamins are absorbed by fat and thus can be stored in the body. Water-soluble vitamins are excreted each time we eliminate and thus remain in the body for only a few hours.

Vitamin A is a fat-soluble vitamin essential to growth, reproduction, and maintenance of skin tissue. It is also necessary for maintaining good vision and strong bones and teeth. The main problem with vitamin A is that, though we generally ingest enough of it, we cannot absorb it properly. Vitamin A needs a diet of at least 7 percent fat to be properly metabolized. It also needs adequate amounts of vitamin E so that it is not oxidized and thus destroyed. If you have been under stress (and what new mother hasn't?) or have had a recent infection or virus, such as a simple cold, most of your vitamin A supply will have been exhausted. U.S. government surveys indicate that one third of all women and as many as 50 percent of our children have some form of vitamin A deficiency. Vitamin A deficiencies are often difficult to recognize, since only a few of us manifest such overt symptoms as temporary blindness. Other symptoms may include dry skin and digestive disorders. The best sources of vitamin A are fish-liver oils. These oils do not taste good, but they are practically calorie-free, as opposed to other vitamin A sources, such as butter and ice cream. Other good sources of vitamin A include carrots, peaches, yams, tomatoes, and squash; 25,000 international units (or I.U.) of natural vitamin A meets the daily adult requirement. This is of course assuming that both you and your breast-fed baby are in good health. If not, your requirements may be higher. There has been a great deal of publicity on vitamin A toxicity. Most of this toxicity, however, has been caused by synthetic preparations—man-made chemical preparations—not natural derivatives, which essentially are concentrated natural foods. Natural foods generally contain a modest amount of a given nutrient, certainly never enough to cause harm to an individual, providing he is not allergic to this particular food. Chemicals, on the other hand, have to be administered with care, as they are more likely to cause disturbances than is natural food. Synthetic products which contain as much as 500,000 I.U. of vitamin A, as opposed to the 25,000 I.U. that are the recommended intake, have caused headaches, drowsiness, loss of hair, and vomiting. If your diet is rich in natural vitamin A sources, you will not need any chemical preparations. Also, beware of the mineral oils contained in some lotions and creams. When you rub these products on your body, vitamin A is actually dissolved, passed into your blood, and eliminated in your feces!

The vitamin B group is probably the most difficult set of nutrients to obtain in the typical American diet, and yet the B vitamins are perhaps the most valuable nutrients to the postpartum mother. If you are breast-feeding your child, their value is unsurpassed. Vitamin B was originally thought of as a single vitamin. Now it is seen as an entire family. Since this family exists together in nature, it is almost impossible to be deficient in just a single B vitamin. The B group consists of B_1, B_2, B_6, B_{12}, niacin (B_3), pantothenic acid, folic acid, PABA (para-aminobenzoic acid), biotin, choline, and inositol. All of these vitamins are essential to the new mother for producing energy and for utilizing fats, protein, and carbohydrates. They are also important to the breast-fed infant, to ensure normal brain-cell development.

The reason most postpartum mothers are deficient in the B vitamins is simple. Foods rich in vitamin B are ill-liked: the most common examples are liver, brewer's yeast, and wheat germ. Also, the action of the B vitamins is what is termed "synergistic," meaning that they must work together. Simply going out and buying a bottle of one kind of vitamin B is not going to help; you need all of the B vitamins, in the correct proportions, for them to be assimilated properly. The vitamin B group, being water-soluble, is not stored in the body. The body loses the B vitamins during elimination and also when you are under stress. Thus, the vitamin B group needs to be replenished often.

How much vitamin B do you need? Unfortunately, the statistics vary widely. It is usually determined, however, by your height, your weight, and the amount of sugar and alcohol you normally ingest. How do you know if you may have a vitamin B deficiency? It is safe to say that a majority of postpartum mothers do. The fatigue, irritability, loss of hair, skin problems, and depression so symptomatic in new mothers can be attributed to vitamin B deficiency as well as to hormonal imbalances and emotional stress. The nutritionist Adelle Davis believed that all the discomforts during pregnancy and the postpartum period could be traced directly to vitamin B deficiencies. I am not sure I agree entirely, but a teaspoon of brewer's yeast or powdered desiccated liver in an eight-ounce glass of juice once or twice a day will certainly improve your disposition and the quality of your breast milk. If this is totally unpalatable for you, eat yogurt mixed with wheat germ and unsweetened preserves instead. This preparation is not as rich in the B group as is the yeast or liver powder, but you will enjoy it more and as a result eat it more regularly. *Note:* It is never going to taste good, but it can be tolerated. Also, if your body is unaccustomed to yeast, you may get gas from it at first.

Vitamin C may well be our most popularly taken vitamin, yet because it is water-soluble, you may not be receiving an adequate supply. Since stress significantly increases the need for vitamin C, most doctors would agree that a daily vitamin C supplement of 500 milligrams is in order for almost every postpartum mother. Vitamin C is utilized more completely when taken in conjunction with a flavone compound known as a bioflavonoid, which is part of the vitamin C family and a natural complement to vitamin C. Bioflavonoids are plentiful in the white portion of an orange peel. Have an orange daily and peel it so that some of the white orange peel is still on the orange. Other good sources of vitamin C are lemons, grapes, currants, plums, grapefruit, apricots, cherries, and rosehips. Though there are few cases of scurvy in the United States today, an adequate vitamin C supply can relieve you of other vitamin C deficiency symptoms, such as allergies, infection, bleeding gums, diarrhea, and exhaustion.

Commonly known as the "sunshine vitamin," vitamin D is formed when ultraviolet rays from the sun interact with an oily substance, known as ergosterol, on your skin's surface. When vitamin D is created on the skin during this process, it is absorbed into your skin and then into your bloodstream. Vitamin D is necessary for adequate bone and dental development and maintenance. It prevents muscular weakness and aids in calcium absorption. If you are breast-feeding your child, it can ensure him of a healthy skeletal structure and strong teeth, resistant to decay. Unfortunately, the two best and perhaps the only reliable sources of this vitamin are the sun and fish-liver oils. The problem with using the sun as a source is that we generally spend too much time indoors, especially in colder climates. When we do get "our day in the sun," we overdo it and perhaps expose ourselves to the dangers of skin cancer. The less dangerous result of overexposure to the sun is dry skin and very little vitamin D absorption (since we tend to shower after a day at the beach, thereby washing off all of the vitamin D we have accumulated). The problem with fish-liver oils, like some other nutritious foods, is that to many people they are not palatable. Next to the sun and to fish-liver oils, egg yolks are the best source of vitamin D. I prefer taking fish-liver-oil capsules; that way you don't have to taste anything. Lack of vitamin D can result in insomnia, muscle spasms, cavities, and nosebleeds. Vitamin D requirements range from 400 I.U. to 50,000 I.U. daily. This wide range may indicate that at present there is not substantial data upon which to base a recommendation.

Out of all the vitamins to be included in the postpartum diet, vitamin E has been the most neglected. Like the B vitamins, vitamin E has been virtually lost due to food refinement. Though this vitamin will not make you more sexy, as commercials claim (though it may give you the energy to enjoy more sexual activity), it will increase the oxygen available to the heart and other muscles and thus improve your circulation. It also heals and protects your reproductive organs, prevents and heals varicose veins, prevents anemia, and relieves leg cramps.

Though studies are still incomplete at this writing, vitamin E has been connected to cancer prevention, especially those cancers associated with female disorders (for example, breast, cervical, and uterine cancer). Very basically, the sluggishness, body ache, and general fatigue that accompany postpartum recovery can be greatly reduced, and in some cases eliminated, by including 400 I.U. (less than a fraction of an ounce) of vitamin E daily. Since the richest sources of vitamin E, which include vegetable oils and whole-grain cereals, are so highly refined commercially, it may be easiest for you to meet your daily vitamin E requirement in the form of capsules of wheat-germ oil or other vitamin E sources. Otherwise, you can choose to eat natural, unprocessed wheat germ, which is easily purchased at any health-food store. Peanuts, eggs, sunflower seeds, and soybeans are also good sources of vitamin E.

Women with high blood pressure or a rheumatic heart condition, however, should restrict their vitamin E intake to about 150 I.U. per day, since a larger dose than this tends to raise the blood pressure. And no one should take more than 800 I.U. of vitamin E daily without a doctor's explicit instructions. Also, vitamin E and the mineral iron should not be taken together, as these chemical compounds tend to cancel each other out. Since vitamin E is fat soluble, it can be stored in the body.

Another fat-soluble vitamin is vitamin K. Women don't worry too much about this vitamin, mainly because its deficiency is often not apparent. Vitamin K's main contribution to life support is normal blood clotting. Vitamin K promotes the manufacture of thrombin, the clotting factor. The lochia and the discomfort that generally accompanies it can be greatly reduced by eating foods rich in vitamin K. Since your intestinal tract manufactures vitamin K, 20 to 25 milligrams of this vitamin daily is sufficient. Problems may arise because this vitamin is easily destroyed. Simply eating frozen food, using mineral oil, or taking an aspirin tablet can destroy substantial amounts of vitamin K. However, if you make yogurt or alfalfa sprouts a regular part of your daily diet, you can be sure to replenish the needed supply. Large doses of this vitamin used to be injected into the laboring mother in the hopes of preventing cerebral palsy in her newborn infant. The vitamin, however, was administered in synthetic form and proved to be toxic. Vitamin K in its man-made form is no longer available without a prescription.

Minerals, like vitamins, are also responsible for the regulation of body fluids and the balance of chemicals in the body. One fact that may surprise you is that minerals are actually more important to your body than vitamins. Vitamins assist in the absorption of minerals but, without minerals, vitamins would have no function The body can manufacture some vitamins, but it cannot manufacture minerals. We must get our minerals from the foods we eat.

The mineral found in the greatest amount in the body is calcium. The average woman has about two to three and a half pounds of calcium in her body. Ninety-nine percent of this is in the bones and teeth. Improper absorption of calcium is the main reason for calcium deficiencies, and not merely inadequate calcium ingestion. Calcium is absorbed in acid and fat. If a woman does not eat adequately during her pregnancy, very little acid will be produced in her intestinal tract, and most of her calcium will be expelled in her feces. Insufficient assimilation of calcium can cause tooth decay, gum disease, cramps, nervousness, and insomnia. Most nutritionally oriented physicians recommend at least 1100 milligrams (sometimes 2000 milligrams) of calcium during postpartum recovery. There is no need to worry about taking too much calcium. If you do, it is merely stored in your long bones for future use or excreted. If you are worried about calcium deposits, it is wise to note that abnormal deposits arise from multiple nutritional deficiencies and not from eating too much calcium. In other words, if you are eating a balanced diet, you don't need to concern yourself. However, if you are suffering from several nutritional deficiencies, then calcium deposits may be the result. If you are concerned, always consult your physician.

Though you can obtain good supplies of calcium from yogurt, cheese, broccoli, and whole grains, I still recommend bone meal and powdered egg shell (one egg shell has 1700 milligrams of calcium and practically no calories). I recommend them because they provide such an excellent balance of calcium, phosphorus, and vitamin D. These products can be purchased in most health-food stores. They come in mint-flavored tablets or in preparations to be mixed with juice or milk. Phosphorus is also present in substantial amounts in the body. Phosphorus works in conjunction with calcium but is contained in more foods (meat and cheeses) and thus there is rarely a phosphorus deficiency.

The role of magnesium is similar to that of calcium, though magnesium is connected more with nerve functions within the brain than with skeletal structure, as is calcium. Even a mild deficiency in magnesium can cause sensitivity to noise, trembling, and depression. Since, as a postpartum mother, you are particularly susceptible to emotional upheaval, doctors recommend about 500 milligrams of magnesium daily. This, fortunately, is rather simple to obtain from green leafy vegetables, nuts, whole grains, and beans. If you choose wisely from these food groups, your magnesium supply should be more than sufficient.

Sodium and chlorine (see my discussion on salt on page 68) are overused by the average American. Sodium and chlorine maintain water balance and muscular functions. In order to keep fluids in the body and to prevent them from being constantly eliminated during urination, a minimum amount of salt is needed. In hot weather salt may need to be replaced more often, due to frequent perspiration, but in general, large amounts of salt (of which sodium and chlorine are components) are not recommended.

Potassium works with sodium to maintain water balance and aids in maintaining heart rhythm. The most common indication of a potassium deficiency is muscular weakness. Fortunately, there are many potassium-rich foods available to you. Potassium is contained in meat, fish, dried fruit, raw vegetables, molasses, bananas, and sunflower seeds. You, as a postpartum mother, should note that the added stress (stress depletes potassium) of your condition and of your new duties may deplete your potassium supply, and therefore you may need to replenish it more often than you might expect.

Though only 0.2 milligrams of iodine are necessary daily, this small amount can prevent goiter, anemia, and weight gain; a portion of seafood or the moderate use of iodized salt can prevent these conditions.

Even if you took an iron supplement religiously during your pregnancy, and though only 10–18 milligrams of iron are necessary per day, anemia is still fairly common among pregnant and postpartum women. Before pregnancy, anemia is usually due to the process of menstruation, in which many red blood cells, containing iron, are lost. During pregnancy, anemia is due to the fetus's red-blood-cell requirement. During the three to six weeks of postpartum lochia, the loss of red blood cells again occurs. Another reason anemia is common, despite an excellent diet, is that the body has difficulty absorbing iron. Good supplies of both vitamin C and vitamin E are necessary to assimilate iron. (*Note:* As I mentioned earlier, iron and vitamin E cancel each other out. This does not mean that they are not needed by the system. Vitamin E should be already present in the system for iron to be absorbed. If iron is not properly assimilated by the presence of vitamin E, it is eliminated from the body in the feces.) Though meat, eggs, whole-grain breads, cereals, wheat germ, and liver are excellent sources of iron, most physicians and nutritionists favor iron supplementation. The reasoning for this is simple. If you eat all of the food necessary for the proper absorption of iron—that is, to obtain the 10–18 milligrams per day which are necessary but which would generally require the consumption of several pounds of meat or their equivalent—you are apt to become extremely overweight. Go to the health-food store and get a natural supplement. In this way, you will prevent the fatigue and listlessness that may accompany an iron-poor diet.

I have listed the most important minerals, but there are many more—manganese, zinc, chromium, selenium, copper, lithium, and cobalt are all trace elements which the body requires to function properly. The body's requirements of these minerals have not yet been established. Supplementation of these trace minerals, above the amounts found in wholesome foods, should not be undertaken without consulting a physician well versed in nutrition. All of these minerals are contained in healthy supplies in fresh fruit and vegetables.

Though, in many cases, I have suggested vitamin and mineral supplements in my previous discussion, I want to emphasize that ideally all vitamins and minerals should be obtained by eating natural foods. Most physicians and nutritionists would agree with this view. Natural sources are always more beneficial to the body than are their chemical equivalents. One hundred years ago, eating natural foods may not have been difficult, but today very few of us have our own cow or can grow our own vegetables. Therefore I recommend a moderate amount of supplementation merely to bridge the gap between good nutrition and the non-nutritional processed foods that you may occasionally eat. In many cases, supplementation is more convenient. A postpartum mother simply does not have the time to count milligrams all day long. A well-balanced food supplement can do that for you, and it's crucial to have the best possible nutrients for your body.

If whipping unfamiliar vitamins and protein substances in your blender and swallowing cod-liver oil seem peculiar to you, believe me that I felt the same way when I began to supplement my diet eight years ago. But now I can say whatever ailments I may have suffered from in the past have either vastly improved or entirely disappeared. My teeth and gums are healthier, my hair is thicker, and my muscles feel stronger. Remember, natural-food supplements (as opposed to synthetic vitamins and minerals) are just plain food in a more concentrated form. While they do not offer overnight miracles, they are extremely important to your health. A healthful diet during postpartum recovery will vastly improve your physical well-being as well as your mental well-being.

There are a few final points I wish to make here. Unless it

is explicitly prescribed by your physician, do not take medication of any kind if you choose to breast-feed your baby. Drugs can be toxic to both you and your breast-fed infant. If you need a simple laxative, rather than using a chemical preparation, try a teaspoon of herbs or a cup of herbal tea before going to bed. It will restore your regularity gently and naturally.

Though no single food is going to provide you with complete nutrition, there are some high-power foods or their derivatives that provide greater nutritional value than most others. Lecithin, a soybean derivative, is an example. This substance is found in every cell in the body, especially in the brain. Lecithin absorbs excess fat and redistributes body weight evenly. (See the section "The Scourge of Cellulite" in this chapter.) Lecithin is nature's tranquilizer because it coats the myelin sheath that surrounds nerve endings. Medical journals indicate that lecithin may be effective in treating gallstones. Lecithin contains protein and almost every vitamin and mineral of essential value. Two tablespoons of lecithin daily—either powdered, liquid, or granule, or the capsule equivalent—can do wonders for you.

Of all foods that have been nutritionally tested, alfalfa has proved to be one of the most nutritionally complete. It is plentiful in both vitamins and minerals and contains every essential amino acid. It has been found, in some cases, to prevent disease and relieve such ailments as bursitis and arthritis. In addition to this, it is a natural diuretic that can virtually eliminate water retention. You may either eat alfalfa as sprouts in your salad or take it in tablet form.

Other potent foods include wheat germ, brewer's yeast, sunflower seeds, and liver. Though they may not seem the most appetizing foods, I suggest you try to include as many of them as possible in your weekly menus, since their nutritional value is high while their comparable caloric count is low.

The preparation of your food is also important. Eat fresh, raw foods as often as possible. Though cooked food is not always detrimental, heating food in general may rob the food of some nutritional value. Steam your vegetables instead of boiling them. To ensure that the vitamins and minerals in your vegetables are still intact, stop steaming your vegetables when they are slightly hard, and not soft or mushy. Use herbs and spices rather than salt for seasoning. (See more on food substitutions in the section "Losing That 'Baby Fat,'" in this chapter.) Meats and fish should be poached and broiled in their own juices rather than fried. Beware of gravies, sauces, and salad dressings; make sure they are prepared from natural sources, without saturated fats or starches.

Perhaps the single factor that calls for a healthful, balanced postpartum diet the most is stress. Stress constantly robs the body of vital nutrients. Modern living has created a tremendously tense society. Being a new mother and having the responsibilities of being a loving wife, a concerned mother, and a diligent career woman can at times be overpowering. When your body is working for you, however, the tensions of daily life can be greatly reduced. Remember that eating correctly and sensibly is important not only for you but for your baby. Having a grouchy, fatigued mother is not fun! Whether or not you have been conscientious about your diet during your pregnancy, postpartum recovery is a time to reevaluate seriously your eating habits and learn to maintain a good nutritional program for a lifetime of health and energy.

THE SCOURGE OF CELLULITE

One method of making money is to coin a fancy word for a common condition and then manufacture a "cure" for it. Cellulite, or *peau d'orange* (orange-peel skin), is one such sham. Cellulite is fat—not fancy fat or French fat. Researchers from Johns Hopkins Medical School have examined both regular fat and what has been termed "cellulite" under the microscope and found their cellular structures to be identical. Cellulite is not toxic, as some may have led you to believe, but has caused great concern among women.

Cellulite is almost exclusively a female condition. Women have a greater percentage of fat in their bodies than men do and are thus more predisposed to accumulating excess fat. "But why are my fatty deposits lumpy and a man's fatty deposits smooth?" a woman may ask. A man's adipose structure is different from a woman's. The fat in a man's body forms in sheets, while a woman's forms in globular postules. Woman's adipose cells are larger and farther apart than a man's. This results in the cottage-cheese texture of cellulite.

Even if you have been fortunate enough to avoid cellulite in your early life, pregnancy and the postpartum period can cause it to develop. The processes of pregnancy and lactation cause excess fatty tissue to accumulate in your body, and unless you are rigid in maintaining your daily exercise program, cellulite will inevitably appear.

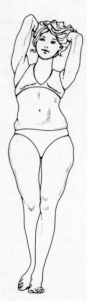

Places in the body most prone to cellulite

The most common places for cellulite to accumulate are your thighs, your buttocks, and the backs of your upper arms. Even if you return to your ideal weight, the cellulite that has formed in these areas may cling to you relentlessly. Why this is so is not completely understood. One theory is that, as child-bearing women, we need extra fatty stores surrounding our pelvic areas to protect the pelvis and the vital reproductive organs. However, since cellulite is merely ordinary fat, it does respond to diet and exercise. It will not respond to creams, magic pills or plastic heat wraps. Massage has been implicated in helping to redistribute fatty cells, but this remains to be proved. The claims of some of the cellulite treatments are very misleading if not outright fallacious.

If you do have excess accumulations of cellulite, examine your diet carefully. (See the previous section in this chapter.) Are you eating too much junk food? Are you frying rather than broiling or baking your meat and poultry? If so, eliminate these practices or at least greatly reduce them. Drink plenty of water (at least eight glasses per day) and include lecithin in your diet. Lecithin is a fat emulsifier that helps to distribute body fat more efficiently. If you have a great deal of cellulite, you may have to lose three to five pounds below your normal weight. *Note:* Excessive reducing strategies are not recommended if you are breast-feeding a baby. Always consult your doctor.

The worst enemy of cellulite is not a good diet. It is exercise (see Chapter Three). Thigh and buttock exercises are extremely effective, but so is walking. When you walk you utilize the very muscles prone to cellulite. So walk whenever you can. Take a good, brisk fifteen-minute walk every day. This continued practice can bring about incredible results.

LOSING THAT "BABY FAT"

Though I have discussed various methods to encourage weight loss in this chapter, I want to emphasize that there is no secret method to weight maintenance. Dieting is not good enough. Anyone can diet and lose weight. The tough part is keeping it off permanently. Weight loss and weight maintenance during the postpartum period is not simple. But keeping that excess weight indefinitely can result in difficulties in your subsequent pregnancies. If you are overweight, it means your eating habits are not good. Other animals in their natural habitat do not become overweight, because they eat only when they are hungry. As I've stressed, eating only when you are hungry and eating only good, nutritious food are the two best eating habits you can develop.

The following information is given only as a guideline. You know what you should weigh and what you would like to weigh. You know at what weight you feel the most comfortable. The sample menu is only a suggestion. In the end you, with your physician's advice, must decide what is best for you.

"HOW MUCH SHOULD I WEIGH?"

The following is a chart developed by the Metropolitan Life Insurance Company. It outlines the desirable weights for women over the age of twenty-five. If you are breast-feeding, you may add three to five pounds to obtain your ideal weight.

	Small Frame	Medium Frame	Large Frame
4′ 11″	99	105	112
5′ 0″	100	107	114
5′ 1″	102	109	116
5′ 2″	105	112	119
5′ 3″	108	115	122
5′ 4″	111	119	126
5′ 5″	114	122	128
5′ 6″	118	125	133
5′ 7″	121	129	137
5′ 8″	124	132	140
5′ 9″	128	136	144
5′ 10″	131	140	147
5′ 11″	134	142	150

Note: You may be slightly above or below the suggested weights and still be quite healthy. Check with your doctor to determine what is the ideal weight for you.

SAMPLE MENU AND FOOD SUBSTITUTION CHART

I have organized this menu in minimeal fashion, as I find it is the most helpful to postpartum mothers. If you are *not* breast-feeding, eat about 300–500 calories less than the list suggests. This particular diet provides between 1700 and 2000 calories per day. If you are not truly hungry for any of these meals, do not eat them just because they are on the list. You may make any intelligent food substitutions. Again, check with your doctor before you commence any new dieting regimen.

BREAKFAST

Blender preparation: whip in blender ½ cup milk *or* ½ cup apple juice, 1 egg, and 1–2 teaspoons of a combined mixture of soybean powder and brewer's yeast

1 orange *or* ½ grapefruit *or* 1 4-ounce glass tomato juice

Suggested vitamin and mineral supplements

1 capsule of vitamins A and D (A—10,000 I.U.; D—400 I.U.)

1 B-complex vitamin tablet (500 milligrams)

1 vitamin C tablet (500 milligrams)

1 vitamin E capsule (400 I.U.)

MID-MORNING

½ cup yogurt with sprinkle of wheat germ and with fresh fruit

¼ cup oatmeal (or any other whole-grain cereal) with 4 ounces milk and sprinkle of raisins or other dried fruit

LUNCH

3 ounces seafood, chicken, or lean meat *or* ½ cup cottage cheese *or* 1 cup fresh vegetable or bean soup *or* 1 teaspoon peanut butter on 1 slice whole-grain bread *or* ½ cup brown rice with ½ cup steamed vegetables (if you have this, you don't need the salad)

½ cup salad (may include romaine or other types of lettuce, tomato, zucchini, alfalfa sprouts, bean sprouts) with salad dressing made with unsaturated oil and vinegar

After lunch:

multimineral tablet including calcium (1100 mg); magnesium (500 mg); iodine (.2 mg); iron (18 mg)

if desired:

1 slice whole-grain bread
1 8-ounce glass milk
herbal tea or coffee substitute

MID-AFTERNOON

1 slice cheese *or* piece of fresh fruit *or* homemade bran or corn muffin *or* homemade oatmeal cookie

DINNER

3 ounces lean meat, chicken, or seafood
4 ounces fresh or cooked vegetables
fresh fruit dessert

if desired:

½ cup brown rice
1 small baked potato
1 slice whole-grain bread
1 8-ounce glass milk
herbal tea or coffee substitute

BEDTIME

if desired:

same blender preparation as you had for breakfast
herbal tea

FOOD SUBSTITUTION CHART

Instead of	*Have*
sugar	fructose, date sugar, honey, natural maple syrup
salt	sea salt, kelp, herbs and spices
white flour	whole-grain flours
saturated oils	unsaturated oils: e.g., safflower, soybean, sesame
red meat	chicken, seafood, meat substitutes such as soybeans
carbonated sodas	natural carbonated mineral water, cider, fruit juices
canned/frozen vegetables	fresh vegetables
processed cheese food	natural cheese with enzymes
chocolate	carob powder
coffee	coffee substitutes made from grains
tea	herbal tea
sour cream	yogurt
ice cream	frozen yogurt

TAKING CARE OF YOURSELF

It is important for you, as a postpartum mother, to do everything possible to make yourself feel better. A simple thing like taking a nap or having a new haircut will do wonders for your disposition. Once a week, have a beauty hour (independently of your exercise time). Use this time to do something special for yourself. The following are a few suggestions.

"I AM SO TIRED." COPING WITH FATIGUE

Because lack of sleep is the single most common complaint from postpartum mothers, I have devoted a section to fatigue. There seems, at first, to be no escape from it. No matter how much rest a woman has during her pregnancy, she is never adequately prepared for the nocturnal habits of the newly born.

To understand fully the significance of this issue, it's helpful to examine the nature of sleep itself. Until twenty-five years ago, there had been little research on sleep and its relationship to the development of personality. Of course, the phenomenon of dreams has been discussed and analyzed since biblical times. Freud and his followers introduced an entire system of psychoanalysis based partly on individuals' dreams as manifestations of the subconscious. But dreaming, though significant, is only a small part of the process of sleep.

Sleep disorders in themselves are criteria for recognizing depression. Almost all people suffering from clinical depression (depression that has been identified professionally) manifest some sleeping disturbances. Though the depressed person may in some instances sleep incessantly, the most common pattern is different. The depressed person will not be able to fall asleep immediately; he or she will remain awake for an hour or two, tossing and turning. When he does fall asleep, he does not experience the deeply satisfying slumber necessary to rejuvenate the mind and the body. The sleep is a kind of peripheral sleep—like a catnap. The person remains in this condition for approximately three to four hours and then pops up as if injected with a strong stimulant. This usually occurs during the small hours of the morning. He is unable to return to sleep at this point and generally busies himself with small chores.

How does this relate to postpartum depression? One young woman describes it quite well.

For the first eight weeks my baby ate every two hours, day and night. Though people told me to nap during the day, I couldn't. It was more difficult for me to wake up after a short rest rather than just stay awake. Besides, I became anxious about housework. The only time I could do the dishes or vacuum was when my baby was asleep. When he was awake he wanted to eat. Since I was breast-feeding, my body adapted to the feedings every two hours. If he somehow skipped a feeding, which was rare, my breasts would be swollen and sore until he was ready to eat again. At night, I did try to sleep, but one ear was always cocked to listen for his cries. Slowly he began to give up certain feedings. He would actually sleep from two A.M. to six A.M., sometimes seven A.M. This sounds great. I was finally able to get five hours of sleep all at once. But I wasn't. I don't know if I was still anxious that he would want that four A.M. feeding or whether I was so used to being awake at that hour, but for two months after he surrendered his four A.M. feeding, I was up at four A.M. and I couldn't get back to sleep. I had never had insomnia before, and what a time to get it — when I needed my sleep the most!

This story is not uncommon. I have had women tell me that they didn't sleep well for the first year after their child's arrival. The newborn has no conception of day and night. He has been comfortably nestled in a warm, dark womb for nine months. When he embarks into this new world, he has to learn about new waking and sleeping hours. The average newborn eats every two hours if he is breast-fed. If he is bottle-fed, he will eat every four hours. This is because mother's milk can be digested more quickly than infant formula. A very young breast-feeding child may wake up and feed from twenty to forty-five minutes, fall asleep for one and a half hours, and then feed again. The infant is actually sleeping a great deal— from twelve to sixteen hours per day. The problem is that he is sleeping for incredibly short intervals.

So it is not the amount of sleep you may theoretically be able to get that will disturb you. It is the interruption of sleep. No one enjoys being awakened in the middle of the night. Scientists have conducted numerous experiments on this phenomenon. Subjects who were interrupted at regular intervals became cranky, irritable, disoriented, and even psychotic. Their control-group counterparts—even if they were deprived of a few hours' sleep, perhaps awakened earlier than they were

accustomed but still allowed a full six to eight hours of uninter-
rupted sleep—functioned on a much higher level.

Fortunately, this traumatic period of sleeplessness tends to
taper off within six to eight weeks after childbirth. The newborn will have adjusted to longer sleeping intervals by then.
Instead of requesting four feedings per night, he may be satisfied with two. However, you can expect to be up at least once
during the night for the first year. And with today's approach
now leaning toward demand feeding rather than the scheduled
feedings suggested thirty years ago, there is greater need for
flexibility on the part of the mother.

The fatigue cycle, however, can become a self-perpetuat-
ing one, especially if you do not take care of yourself. When
you are fatigued, you become more irritated by chores and
projects left undone. Things that didn't bother you before can
suddenly seem to be very important. You may try to overcom-
pensate for this inadequate feeling by doing too much. As a
result, you become too tired to eat properly and the effect of
poor nutrition brings an even greater fatigue. And, due to the
continuing stress of fatigue, you crawl into bed at night and
find you can't fall asleep.

When this happens, there are several things you can do to
offset it. First, take ample amounts of the vitamin B-complex.
The B family of vitamins, like vitamin C, are stress-reducing
vitamins. Once you are more relaxed, you may be able to forget irrelevant matters and eat adequately. Make the two hours
before you go to sleep as peaceful as possible. Unless they are
pressing, leave the office duties and the household chores alone
during this time. Go to bed about a half hour before you plan
to go to sleep, and read, watch television, or listen to comforting music. Don't eat too much or drink anything stimulating
before you retire. Regular daily exercise, though not recommended immediately before bedtime, can also relieve fatigue.

Remember that the first six to eight weeks of new motherhood will naturally be marked by fatigue. One thing to remember is not to persecute yourself for this. Many women feel inad-

equate during this time, as if they felt they were not strong enough to be mothers. Fortunately, the body and the mind gradually adapt, but not without complication and compromise. If you succumb to stress and fatigue, you are reacting in a perfectly natural way to a natural phenomenon.

"AM I GOING BALD?" YOUR HAIR

During your pregnancy, your hair gleamed and thickened. Any previous hair problems seemed to disappear, destined never to return. Your placenta and the rich proteins it housed were largely responsible for your lustrous mane. Once your placenta is expelled, you no longer have adequate protein in your system to support the previously enormous hair growth, and so your hair begins to fall out. (Hormone imbalance and the stress of new motherhood may also contribute to hair loss.)

This hair-thinning phenomenon is actually quite relative. The average person's hair falls out at approximately 100 strands per day. It's likely that this rate of attrition lessened during your pregnancy but not enough to be truly significant. It is just that the growth of hair during pregnancy is so extreme that we don't miss the lost hair. Normally our hair grows one half inch per month. During pregnancy, it may grow as much as an inch. During the postpartum period you may lose 50–100 percent more hair daily than before you became pregnant. And you will not always have to brush your hair to loosen this thinning hair. You will actually begin to shed—finding hair on your pillow in the morning, or on various articles of clothing.

This, of course, can be very distressing, but there are methods of remedying this. The most basic way is to concentrate on protein foods in your diet. Hair is almost exclusively protein in composition.

Your hair may also tend to be dry and brittle. (It could also become overoily, but this is not common.) If this is the case, take a serious look at the shampoo you are using. If it is detergent-based, it can strip your hair of the vital oils so necessary to moisturizing dry hair and cause your scalp glands to work harder to replace these valuable oils. Exchange your detergent-based shampoo for one that is based in cream made of natural proteins and vegetable oils such as wheat-germ oil. You don't need to wash your hair every day. As a matter of fact, this practice is detrimental to your hair. Give your hair a rest. Three or four shampoos a week is plenty.

Choose a good-quality brush and comb. Sharp teeth and bristles can damage hair. Don't use rubber bands or sleep in hair rollers. Both of these practices cause the hair to split and break.

Get into the habit of using a good conditioner after each shampoo. Apply it generously, especially on the ends. This not only helps to moisturize your hair but helps to avoid tangles. Tugging at tangles will also split and break your hair.

Though it may be advantageous to get a good haircut at this time (long hair is heavy and may tug at your hair follicles and also contribute to hair loss), try to avoid other salon treatments. Dyes and permanent waves are simply not a good idea right now. Both of these processes involve burning of the hair with either ammonia- or alkaline-based solutions. This will cause your hair to dry out even more and may cause damage that is difficult to repair. If you really feel that you need a lift, try natural henna. This product will give your hair a reddish tint and add delightful body at the same time. There are also neutral hennas available that add no color whatsoever, but result in incredible luster. Neutral henna is effective for all hair color, including blond, on which tinted henna should not be used. A chamomile herbal rinse after a henna application will brighten dull, lifeless hair.

Avoid using an electric hair dryer. Your hair will become excessively dry if you use a dryer daily during the postpartum period. There are plenty of hairstyles, both long and short, which can accommodate natural drying. Let your hair dry naturally.

If, due to thinning, your hair needs extra volume, try these little "tricks." For short hair: Spray your hair with a little water and massage with a dab of setting lotion. (There are several protein-rich setting products available.) Let dry and brush gently forward from the nape of your neck. Shake your hair loose by tossing your head and then shape your hair by using your fingers. Now your hair is ready to style. It should be light and fluffy, with extra body.

For long hair: Pull your hair on top of your head into a pony tail with a cloth-covered hair fastener (not a rubber band). Spray with water and massage the hair held in the clasp with setting lotion. If you wish, you can wind your hair in those spongy dime-store rollers. Let your hair dry and remove rollers and fastener. Brush your hair gently. Your hair should be very full and bouncy.

Your hair reflects your state of health. A balanced diet and good hygiene can do more than any hair product.

"MY GUMS ARE BLEEDING." YOUR TEETH

As I explained earlier, the average American woman's diet is seriously calcium-deficient. Teeth and bones need calcium to survive. While all bones surrender some of their valuable calcium at a time when there is a deficiency, they do not give up their calcium evenly. Medical researchers at Cornell University have investigated this phenomenon and found that the jawbone, which houses the lower teeth, suffers the greatest loss.

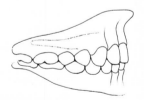

Healthy teeth and gums

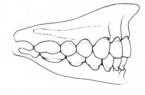

Receded gums

Because both pregnancy and the postpartum period tend to deplete your body's natural calcium supply, you may find that as a result you have inflamed gums and lower incisors turning gray at the roots. In my opinion, and according to experienced, nutritionally minded physicians, bone meal or other calcium supplements are almost essential during the postpartum time, especially if your teeth or gums have been seriously damaged. Vitamin C is also beneficial.

Thorough attention to your teeth and gums at all times and especially during the postpartum period is definitely in order. Brush your teeth twice a day with a soft-bristled brush. Hard bristles can cause gums to bleed. Though some toothpaste is thought to be excellent, sea salt or baking soda is just as useful, is less expensive, and can stimulate the gums more effectively than any toothpaste. If you prefer using toothpaste, choose a brand that includes powdered eggshell (a rich source of calcium). Use dental floss (your dentist can advise you on the correct technique) to dislodge food particles and remove plaque—the bacteria that form on teeth and gums. Another effective method of stimulating your gums is to massage them gently with a soft towel.

Tooth decay and gum disease are the two most universal ailments among Americans. You've got only one set. Be good to them and you will have them for a lifetime.

"MY SKIN IS SO DRY." YOUR SKIN

Though there are many women who may have oily skin during the postpartum period, the vast majority (80–95 percent) lose the natural moisture of their skin. I am not referring just to the skin on your face. Your face represents a small portion of your total body area. The facial area is often of the greatest concern to postpartum women, however, because it is always exposed to nature's drying elements. Whatever your prepregnant skin type, your skin is bound to be a touch drier than you are accustomed to.

Skin dryness is essentially caused by two things: 1) the lack of body fluid and surface moisture and 2) the environment. After childbirth, the chemical substances that ensure proper fluid balance in the body are disturbed by hormone production. If you breast-feed, you are more susceptible to dry skin than if you choose not to nurse. The reason for this is fundamental: Your body is using all available body fluids for milk production.

The most basic remedy is to drink plenty of fluids (two quarts daily—water and fruit juices are best). Whatever moisture you are losing due to hormone imbalance and milk production can be replenished in this manner. This is rarely enough, unfortunately. Dry skin most often requires surface treatment as well.

One of the best surface treatments is a nice steamy bath. Beware of the "sudsy" bubble baths; these often contain detergents and perfumes that will further dry your skin. Instead use an emollient that includes protein, vitamin E, and scent from finely ground herbs. Steep in your bath for about fifteen minutes (longer may be relaxing, but is unnecessary) with a wet towel draped over your face. When you step out, have a good moisturizing lotion available to apply to those problem dry areas—the knees, elbows, buttocks, feet, and hands. (Note: If you need to shave, do so before your bath. Don't use soap or shaving cream. Most of these products are notorious for their drying effects. Instead use a good moisturizer or even your protein-based shampoo.) Don't rub your body dry. Buff it! Take your towel (make sure it is a soft towel), as if you were going to give your body a "shoe shine." Hold it taut between your hands and buff your body dry. This practice actually finishes your skin and makes it gleam with moisturizing oil without leaving that greasy feeling all over your body. (Note: If you are nursing your child, be sure any oil or fragrance is removed from your areolae and nipples before feeding.)

Pay attention to your face. If you have been meticulous in your diet, including all of the valuable nutrients I discussed earlier in this chapter, you should have a minimum of problems, if any. Cleanse your face thoroughly with a protein-based formula. Protein promotes skin elasticity and resiliency. Moisturize generously, especially around the eyes, with a product rich in vitamin E, such as apricot-seed oil and grapeseed oil. Leave your moisturizer on for about ten minutes and then gently remove with cotton pads.

If you are particularly adventurous, you might try the following. For dark shadows (caused by those late hours): Whip an egg white and one fourth of a potato (yes, a potato) into a paste in your blender. Place under your eyes and let set for five minutes. Wash off with lukewarm water and pat dry. For wrinkles and dry lines: Puncture two lecithin capsules and mix with an egg white. Dab onto facial lines and leave on for five minutes. Rinse with lukewarm water and pat dry

Once a week give yourself a good herbal mask. The best preparations are made with green clay and can be purchased in most pharmacies and health-food stores. Smooth all over your face and leave on for fifteen minutes. Rinse your face thoroughly.

Whatever you do, do not stay in the sun too long. A sufficient vitamin D supply can be gained in as little as fifteen to twenty minutes of direct sunlight. We all know the dangers of overexposure, yet some of us still continue to bake ourselves in search of the perfect tan. Tanning ages your skin significantly and may expose you to the dangers of skin cancer. If you absolutely must be in the sun, take these precautions. Moisturize your skin with a good sun-screen lotion, preferably one with vitamin E and PABA. Wear sunglasses and keep your head covered. (*Note:* The following is still a controversial technique; it is not harmful, yet some dermatologists argue its necessity. If you know you are going to be out in the sun, say on vacation, it can be helpful to take PABA internally in tablet form. This may protect you from the ill effects of overexposure to the sun.)

The general condition of your skin, like that of your teeth and hair, is a direct reflection of your health. Eat well, exercise, and keep a healthy mental attitude, and your skin will glow as well.

The necessity of proper nutrition and good hygiene during

postpartum recovery can never be understated. They are both absolutely necessary to the new mother's health and mental well-being. It is also necessary for the postpartum mother to understand fully the biological changes which accompany new motherhood, so that postpartum recovery is accepted more and feared less. With this information intact, let us venture on to the next chapter to discover how exercise can both improve your postpartum experience and allow you to make fitness a regular part of your life.

=3=

GETTING BACK INTO SHAPE:
THE VALUE OF EXERCISE

Many of us create excuses for not exercising. Exercise takes too much time, it's boring, or it is just too much of an effort seem to be common complaints. Consequently, we've become a sedentary nation, plagued with lower back pain, high blood pressure, and tension headaches. This, of course, is changing. Due to the prompting of a good many medical professionals, we are becoming more exercise-conscious. According to the *Journal of the AMA*, 30 to 50 percent more Americans are engaging in regular exercise programs than were a mere ten years ago, and more than half of them are women.

Thirty years ago women didn't exercise much after they finished high school. It wasn't ladylike to perspire, much less participate in a competitive sport. Certainly there were female athletes who broke this rule, but these women were the exception. They were few, and their competitive skills were small compared to those of female athletes today.

Perhaps it was the traditionally sedentary view of life that produced generations of women best anesthetized during childbirth. Women who had never engaged in a more rigorous activity than climbing a flight of stairs could never be expected to endure the pains of childbirth. Women who engaged in back-breaking housework did not often exercise the essential muscles used in childbirth. Statistics still prove that a physically active woman is always more prepared for childbirth than a sedentary one. Women who do little exercise before labor often require or request tranquilizers or other extraordinary assistance during delivery.

But what about exercise after childbirth? The same theory holds. If a woman has been physically active, her body will be quick to resume its former shape. If she has not, she will have to begin to apply herself to a serious exercise program. There are several indications that you may need either more exercise or a specific kind of exercise to help you feel like your old self after childbirth: Pounding of the heart after minor exertion such as lifting your baby or vacuuming the living room; stiffening of the legs or thighs after climbing the stairs; and the experience of frequent restlessness or inability to awaken refreshed even after a good lengthy nap are symptoms. If you are experiencing any of these symptoms, do see your doctor. In all likelihood you are in need of a regular exercise program.

How we care for our bodies during our daily activities is just as important as how we support them while we are exercising. The positions we sleep in, the way we walk all reflect the attention we have given ourselves. The following are suggestions on proper care for your body not only during postpartum recovery but for a lifetime.

If the prospect of a new exercise regimen is beginning to sound particularly dreary to you, I don't mean it to be so. Exercise is a kind of religion with me. It is part of my life, like eating or sleeping, and I try to make it as enjoyable as possible. I have known women in their seventies who had never exercised before. When they finally entered exercise programs to relieve some malady or another, they became exercise addicts within six months.

I had such awful posture it made my walking difficult.
Now I stand up, pull in my stomach, and I feel like a new
person. If only someone had told me this fifty years ago.

I hear testimonials like this one constantly from women of
all ages. The first step and the most difficult one, of course, is to
commit yourself. Tell yourself you are going to exercise regularly for the rest of your life. And you are going to have fun
doing it, and feel better. The first step in setting up an exercise
program is to establish a schedule. Choose a fairly consistent
time during which your baby regularly sleeps. For instance,
plan three half-hour periods evenly spaced during the week
when you have hired a baby-sitter—Monday, Wednesday, and
Friday, at 1 P.M. for example. Write your schedule down and
tack it up someplace where you can see it. Even if you are
fatigued, which unquestionably you will be, try not to use this
as an excuse not to exercise. Remember, exercise is going to
stimulate you and make you less tired. After a few weeks of
moderate exercise, you will actually have more energy than
when you began. The benefits of exercise are numerous. You
will acquire stronger muscles, heart, lungs, and circulatory system. You will have more endurance, better coordination, greater joint flexibility, and a reduction of minor aches and pains.
Exercise helps to overcome or prevent emotional tension and in
some cases has helped prevent critical diseases such as heart
disease and stroke. It can improve your posture, relieve constipation, and help you to control your appetite. And to top if off,
it will give you a healthy, well-toned body! It's worth it for a
mere one and a half hours per week.

In preparation, get yourself some comfortable exercise at-
tire and a soft, thick blanket or mat, if you don't like to exercise
on the bare floor. You may exercise to music; some people find
this soothing. I often exercise during a particularly mindless
television program. It makes my evening more interesting.

My own exercise program is very carefully planned. I have
designed it to incorporate all essential body parts, especially

those which have undergone dramatic changes in pregnancy. I begin my program right at the beginning of postpartum recovery, with some general advice, including some exercises you can do in your hospital bed. I then proceed to common-sense practices in the belief that everyday actions such as sitting and walking can actually become a form of exercise when performed correctly.

The next section is my stretching section. Stretching is an essential part of any exercise program. The body must be supple before it can adequately accept more strenuous activity. If you do not stretch before doing more strenuous exercise, you can injure yourself.

Begin with the warm-up exercises which are part of the stretching exercise. The warm-up I will describe here prepares your basic muscle groups for activity. The later exercises are grouped according to specific parts of your body.

The objective or purpose of a given exercise is listed directly under the title of the exercise in the following manner. The primary body part to be exercised is listed first; if there are secondary body parts, they are listed afterward.

In the instructions that follow, I have grouped exercises in order of increasing difficulty—the last exercise listed being the most strenuous of the group. Difficulty, of course, is always a relative matter. There is no reason for you to feel that an exercise which is presented earlier must be more simple than one which is presented later. Everyone's body is different. If you come to an exercise which seems to be impossible for you, do not press yourself at first. Do what you can and go on to the next exercise. The purpose of the program is to stretch and strengthen the body, not to strain it. This rule particularly applies to the number of exercise repetitions. The repetitions I recommend at the conclusion of each exercise are ideals for women in good shape. No one should begin to perform an exercise the maximum number of times; work up to it. Before you begin, always check the section "Suggested Exercise Sequences/Routines" located at the end of Chapter Three, to make sure that you are performing at a level that is commensurate with your ability.

The stretching exercises are often coupled with a controlled form of breathing similar to several yoga practices. Do not become overanxious about this. Controlled breathing helps you to release and elongate muscles—allowing them to stretch more easily and with greater freedom. Employ the following procedure when using controlled breathing. When you inhale, breathe in through your nose and fill both your upper and lower abdomen with air. Exhale through your mouth and pull your stomach in as far as possible. If you need further elaboration, see the breathing exercises in the section "For Relaxation."

In several exercises, I employ "counts." Counting, of course, without a given tempo is going to be subjective. However, what I hope to show by counting is that an exercise which requires two counts will be performed at a much quicker rhythm than one that needs eight counts. If I do not indicate a definite number of counts in a given exercise, it means that counting does not have a direct bearing on that particular exercise. If you can adapt your own personal rhythm to this relative scale, then you will have a general idea of the tempo of any given exercise.

The rotational exercises, which are part of the stretching exercises, are more related to your bone and skeletal structure than your musculature. Your bone structure, primarily in your pelvic girdle and lower back, has also undergone extraordinary changes due to pregnancy and needs special exercise to restore its alignment.

My strengthening exercises are in the next section. They should be performed after the completion of a combination of stretching and rotational exercises. Again, please refer to the section "Suggested Exercise Sequences/Routines" in this chapter for a thorough description of the best exercise format for you. The strengthening exercises are, in general, the most strenuous ones and for maximum benefit should always be worked into gradually.

Before you begin any exercise program, it is essential to check with your doctor. He or she will be best able to determine your capabilities. A conservative medical view allows for the beginning of a moderate exercise program six to eight weeks after delivery. That is, in my opinion, quite conservative. If you were accustomed to rigorous exercise before your pregnancy and maintained a healthy prenatal exercise program, you may be able to resume activity sooner than this.

The most important consideration for you and your doctor is to make certain that you do not have any underlying condition which would contraindicate an exercise program. I strongly suggest that you show this exercise section to your doctor. If he or she feels that certain exercises would not be beneficial in your case, by all means adapt your program accordingly.

Finally, I want to include a note on the philosophic view of exercise. I believe, as the ancient Greeks and Romans did, that exercise is not for the body alone. Recent studies have confirmed that regular exercise promotes the excretion of endorphins—hormones which are known to relieve depressive symptoms, including those involved in postpartum recovery. It offers a mental and emotional release as well. A regular exercise practice can lighten your disposition, relieve stress, and prevent depression. You will find yourself thinking more clearly and having more patience with your family. A sound, healthy body feeds into the rest of your life, making you more productive, more relaxed, and maybe even happier.

General Advice

WHAT TO DO WHILE YOU ARE STILL IN THE HOSPITAL

Many hospitals are now in the habit of giving you a list of exercises to do about twelve to twenty-four hours after delivery. These exercises are necessary to facilitate the return of the uterus to its prepregnancy size. They also help alleviate the sluggishness or incontinence of your elimination processes which often follow delivery. Here are a few simple exercises to do in your hospital bed—with your doctor's consent. Remember, the idea is not to exhaust yourself but to improve your pelvic functions. If you become tired, rest and resume the exercises later. While the following information concerning daily activity is not part of your regular exercise program, it is still helpful to view all physical activity in the context of exercise to achieve maximum fitness benefits.

Sleeping Positions

Your lower back, which has been placed under considerable strain during pregnancy, is possibly the most sensitive area of your body. It is certainly the most subject to stress. Faulty sleeping positions can intensify swayback and result not only in lower-back pain but in numbness, tingling, and pain in the arms and legs. To avoid this lower-back tension, sleep on a firm mattress; this will give your lower back and pelvis the support you need to maintain correct alignment. If your mattress is not firm enough, use a bedboard between the mattress and springs. Never sleep on your stomach. This exaggerates swayback. Do sleep on your back, with a pillow under both of your knees, or on your side with both of your knees bent into a fetal-like position. Both these positions eliminate any spinal curvature you may have and encourage the correct placement of your lower spine and pelvis.

Before getting out of bed in the morning, you may want to try the following. Exercises performed while lying in bed are aimed not so much at strengthening muscles as in teaching the correct positioning for the lower back. Muscles used correctly, however, become stronger and in time are able to support the body with the least amount of effort.

Exercises to Do in Bed

1. Have a pillow folded in half under your neck. Both of your knees are bent, with your feet on the mattress. Bring one of the knees up to your chest and then lower slowly. Do not straighten your legs. Relax. Repeat with each leg ten times.

2. Now bring both of your knees up to your chest. Tighten your abdominal muscles and press your lower back flat against the mattress. Relax. Repeat five times. This exercise gently stretches the shortened muscles of your lower back and pelvis while strengthening your abdominal muscles.

3. Lie on your back, with one leg bent at the knee, the other stretched along the bed. Lift the straight leg a few inches off the bed and lower it slowly. Repeat a half dozen times and then repeat with the other leg. Each time you perform this exercise, try to raise your leg a little higher.

4. Lie on your stomach and turn your head to one side. Arms are at your sides, with the backs of your hands against the mattress. Squeeze your buttock and pelvic muscles gently against each other and hold for a count of four. Rest. Do about ten times.

5. Lie on your stomach, bend your arms at the elbows, and clasp your hands together so that you are able to rest your forehead on the backs of your hands. Bend both knees and lift your buttocks to the ceiling while leaving your chest on the mattress; you will have to slide your upper body closer to your knees to compensate for this position. Make sure your knees are a hip-distance apart (knees in a parallel line with your hips) and that your body weight is concentrated on your chest and not on your arms or legs. Slowly and gently press your abdominal muscles up against your lower back. Hold this position three to five minutes and rest. Repeat twice a day.

SITTING

If you are experiencing any lower-back or pelvic discomfort, sitting is the one thing you should avoid. There are glandular secretions involved in the assimilation of calcium and other mineral substances which become trapped in a seated posture and may cause mineral deposits in your lower spine. Stand properly, as described later in this chapter, or lie down and exercise as I've just described.

If you are ready to sit, choose a firm, straight-back chair.

Soft, lumpy chairs and sofas can never give you the support your lower back requires. When you can, prop your feet up on a footrest. Cross your legs at the ankles, not at the knees. Crossing your legs at the knees interferes with the vital circulation your lower back and reproductive organs require, and may cause varicose veins. Try to keep your neck in a straight line with the rest of your spine and keep your shoulders down. Pull your abdominal muscles flat against your lower back to lift your chest and straighten your back.

STANDING

A straight back and a strong stomach are the essentials for good posture and firm pelvic support. To find your correct standing position, stand one foot away from the wall. Now sit against the wall, bending your knees slightly. Your shoulder blades and buttocks should touch the wall. If only your shoulders touch, you are round-shouldered. If only the middle of your spine touches, your spine is curved too much. Now tighten your abdominal and buttock muscles. This will tilt your pelvis back and flatten your lower spine. Holding this posture, inch up the wall to a standing position by straightening your legs. Now walk around the room (in the same manner described below), maintaining this posture. Return to the wall again and check to see if you have held this posture correctly.

WALKING

All the things your mother told you apply here. Stand tall, shoulders down and relaxed, chest forward, and abdomen pulled flatly against your lower spine. This may sound like a military directive, but it is not rigidness we want to achieve; if your placement is correct, your muscles can be relaxed and still give you maximum support.

A common fault in walking is to tip the head and trunk from side to side. This causes a kind of zigzagging swagger. Since the shortest distance between two points is a straight line, a swinging walk can take you two miles for every one you actually progress, and can place unmentionable strain on the backs of the legs. Legs which do not function properly gradually stiffen up and are unable to provide sufficient support. This muscle strain eventually passes through the legs and into the pelvic area.

To correct this, you must narrow your stance. A majority of people stand with their legs too far apart. Ironically, ballet dancers are the most guilty. Onstage, they are graceful beyond imagination. Offstage, they are forever tripping, falling down, and bumping into people. If only they would learn one thing: to keep their legs underneath them instead of in that exaggerated, turned-out position. Your feet should be in a parallel line with your hips and shoulders. As you walk, you should place one foot directly in front of the other. There is a crisscrossing involved here similar to the gait acquired by a tightrope walker, though his is highly exaggerated. Your foot, when extended forward, should be directly under your shoulder. Step heel down, pressing off with the ball of your foot, and keep your knees relaxed.

This practice will contribute to smoother more graceful walking without fatigue. You will be able to walk greater distances for longer periods of time and create the support for your pelvis you may have previously lacked.

LIFTING

All of us lift objects in the course of the day, and often have to pick up infants and small children. Many lower-back disturbances are caused by improper lifting.

When lifting light packages or your infant, follow these rules: 1) let your legs bear the strain; 2) hold the package or baby as close to your body as possible; 3) keep your back straight; 4) bend from the knees to lift, not the waist. When carrying shopping bags, try to keep the same amount of weight in each hand. This avoids the curving of the spine either to the right or to the left, which may result in the straining of the back or ligaments.

With this general advice in mind, let's go into the specific exercises recommended.

STRETCHING YOUR BODY

Stretching exercises are designed to prepare your body for the more strenuous exercises. They serve to lengthen your muscles, prevent unnecessary strain or injury, avoid muscle spasms, and create flexibility.

**General
stretching**

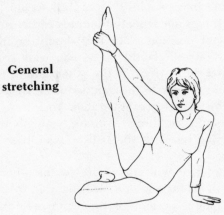

WARMING UP

The following five exercises should always be done prior to any exercise sessions, regardless of your level of proficiency. They prepare essential muscle groups and are especially prescribed if you are unduly stiff or overtired.

Chin to Knee

Purpose: To relax and stretch lower spine and the backs of legs.

Lie flat on your back, with both legs stretched straight along the floor. Now slowly draw your knee up to your chest while simultaneously bringing your chin to your knee. Return to the beginning position. Repeat complete sequence four times. Now repeat the entire exercise using the left leg. Relax.

Now repeat the exercise four times with both legs, bringing your knees up to your chest at the same time.

The Lunge

Purpose: To stretch pelvic floor and inner thighs. (The pelvic floor is a very thin, sheetlike muscle composed of several parts. This muscle provides support for your abdominal cavity, and controls your urine flow and the contractions of your vagina and rectum.)

Kneel down on the floor. Extend your right leg as far to the side as possible, keeping your leg straight and the arch of your foot on the floor. Slide your foot along the floor until you feel the stretch of your inner thigh muscles. Perform this slowly and hold for a count of four. Repeat the exercise, using your left leg.

Arm Crosses

Purpose: To relax upper body and improve circulation.

Stand properly, as described above in "Standing." Raise both of your arms perpendicular to your body and then overhead. Breathe in deeply, and gently swing both arms up over and slightly behind your head. Exhale and drop them down loosely to your sides. Repeat ten times.

Knee Pulls

Purpose: To stretch leg and hip area.

Stand properly, as described before. Bend your right knee and clasp it in front of your body with both hands. Slowly bring your knee as close to your chest as possible and return to the beginning position. (Don't be upset if you lose your balance at first. You will improve with practice.) Complete four times with right leg and then your left leg.

Side Bends

Purpose: To loosen and relax torso.

Stand properly, with the palms of your hands on the outside of your upper thighs. Now slowly bend your torso as far as you can to the right as you slide your right hand down along the side of your right leg. Hold for a slow count of four and return to the beginning position. Complete eight times and repeat on the left side.

YOUR PELVIS

Of all your body parts, your pelvis is definitely the one that has undergone the most extreme changes both structurally and chemically due to the process of pregnancy. It may seem counterproductive to begin to stretch these muscles, which have already been expanded almost beyond their limit. However, the pelvic muscles do need to be stretched and relaxed in order to perform at their optimum. Also, flexible muscles are quite different from flaccid ones. Flexibility enchances the strength and mobility of your pelvic area, whereas flaccid muscles can do nothing to support the vital organs, which are dependent upon firm pelvic support.

The Pelvic Stretch

Purpose: To stretch the pelvic muscles, the lower back, and the inner thighs.

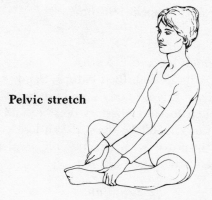

Pelvic stretch

Sit erect on the floor, with your shoulders down into your back. Knees are bent so that the soles of your feet are touching. Your hands are clasping your ankles. Breathe in and allow your stomach to fill with air. Exhale and pull your stomach flat up against your lower back. Allow this action to curl your spine and bring your chin in to your chest. Bring your forehead as close to your heels as possible. Relax in this position. Inhale and exhale four times as your continue to press your stomach up against your lower back. Use your elbows to press your knees closer to the floor. Now breathe in and slowly uncurl your spine until you are in the beginning position. Relax. Do this entire exercise three times.

The Pelvic Floor Stretch

Purpose: To stretch the pelvic floor, inner thighs, and torso.

Sit erect, with your right leg extended on a diagonal on the floor while your left leg is bent into the center of your body in a relaxed position. Extend both arms overhead, elbows straight, but keeping your shoulders down into your back. Breathe in to prepare and, as you exhale, slowly lift and stretch your torso to the right side, keeping a parallel line with your right leg. Breathe in once again and slowly return to your original position. Complete eight times and then repeat the entire exercise with your left leg extended on the diagonal.

The Wide Pelvic Floor Stretch

Purpose: To stretch the pelvic floor, lower back, and torso.

Sit erect, with both of your legs stretched to the side in opposite directions. Extend both arms overhead, elbows straight, being careful to keep your shoulders down into your back. Breathe in to prepare, and exhale, pressing your stomach up against your lower back (as you did in "The Pelvic Stretch"). Bring your chin down in to your chest and reach with both of your arms directly in front of you. Breathe in and return to the beginning position. Complete eight times.

YOUR BACK

Your spine, like your pelvis, has also undergone tremendous strain as a result of your pregnancy. Even those women who previously showed no symptoms of back pain may now feel spinal discomfort. The following exercises, taken from Hatha yoga practice, when performed regularly can provide relief and prepare your back for more strenuous exercise.

The Cobra

Purpose: To stretch and elongate shortened back muscles.

Begin by lying on your stomach, your head turned to one side. Both of your elbows are bent and the palms of your hands are on the floor directly under your shoulders. Breathe in and turn your head face down, and then begin to lift your head off the floor. Exhale and slowly arch your back while using your arms to support yourself. Both of your hip bones should remain on the floor at all times. Keep your chin forward and your eyes upward. When you have arched as fully as you can, breathe in once again and exhale as you slowly lower yourself to the floor and resume your beginning position.

The Bow

Purpose: To limber spinal muscles.

Begin on your stomach, with your neck curved so that the top of your forehead touches the floor. Bend both of your knees, keeping your pelvis on the floor. Reach backward with both of your hands to clasp your ankles. (You may have difficulty with them at first, so take it easy. You may try doing this exercise clasping only one ankle and then progressing to two ankles when you are ready.) Breathe in to prepare, and exhale as you slowly arch your back and pull on your ankles. Your chin is forward and your eyes are looking upward. You may notice a slightly rocking motion in your body due to the pendular position of this exercise. Breathe in once more and exhale as you slowly lower yourself to the floor. Keep your hands clasped about your ankles and complete this exercise four times.

The Plow

Purpose: To limber spine and improve circulation.

Begin lying on your back, with both of your knees bent and your feet flat on the floor. Your arms are bent at the elbows, your palms holding the base of your spine. Bend both of your knees up in to your chest and, using your hands, push your lower body upward and back so that your knees are in a direct line with your head. Now slowly begin to straighten your knees, while supporting your lower back with your hands. If you are limber enough, you may be able to touch your toes to the floor above your head. Now relax in this position, bend your knees slightly, and hold for a count of eight. Slowly uncurl your spine and resume your beginning position. Complete this exercise twice.

The Forward Bend

Purpose: To limber spine and the backs of your legs.

Sit erect, with both of your legs stretched out straight in front of you. Extend both of your arms over your head, keeping your shoulders down into your back. Breathe in to prepare, and exhale as you bring your chin in to your chest and pull your stomach flat against your lower back and reach for your toes with your fingertips. Keep your knees straight and both of your arms in a parallel line to your legs so your elbows are slightly above your ears. Breathe in and resume your beginning position. Complete this exercise eight times.

The Triangle

Purpose: To stretch lower back, hip joints, and the backs of the legs.

Stand with your legs about three feet apart. Bend your torso over from your hips and hang loosely so that your hands can touch the floor. Hold the position for a slow count of four. Twist your torso toward the right leg, clasp your right ankle, and hold for another slow count of four. Now thrust your torso toward your left leg, clasp your left ankle, and hold for a slow count of four. Return your torso to the center and hold for a final four counts. Now slowly uncurl your spine to the standing position. Repeat this exercise once. *Note*: Do not return too abruptly to the standing position, you may become dizzy.

YOUR LEGS

Your legs have been supporting your maternal weight for nine months and may tire easily as a result. They may also be stiff and sore. The following exercises can relieve that tension and prepare your body to reshape those tired muscles.

The "V"

Purpose: To loosen leg and hip muscles.

Lie on your back and bend your knees in to your chest. Straighten your legs so that they form a right angle with your torso. Slowly open your legs to the sides and clasp your hands around your inner thighs for support. Hold this position for a slow count of four and bend your knees. Complete this exercise twice.

Wall Stretching

Purpose: To loosen leg and hip muscles.

Sit facing the wall, the palms of your hands on the floor behind your hips for support. Stretch both of your legs wide so that your toes touch the wall. Your knees should be facing upward toward the ceiling. Slowly, using your hands, begin to push your pelvis toward the wall. Hold this position for a slow count of eight. Repeat this exercise twice.

Long Leg Stretch

Purpose: To stretch the backs of your legs.

Lie on your left side and bend your left arm so that your left hand can support your head. Bend both of your knees so that they form a right angle with your torso. Clasp your right leg with your hand either on the ankle, behind the knee, or in back of the thigh (whichever place is comfortable). Now slowly straighten your knee until your leg is fully extended. Hold this position for a slow count of two and bend your knee. Complete this exercise eight times and then do it with your left leg being extended.

YOUR TORSO AND WAISTLINE

Your torso is perhaps a little "squarer" than before you pregnancy, and that diminutive waistline may seem to have vanished forever. Stretching the torso can help trim your middle and restore your former "hourglass" shape. It also aids circulation.

Standing Side Stretch

Purpose: To loosen hip joints and tighten waistline.

Stand tall, with your feet about three feet apart. Hold your left wrist with your right hand and extend both of your arms overhead. Breathe in to prepare, and exhale as you lift and stretch your torso directly to the right. Inhale and return to the center. Complete this exercise eight times to the right and then reverse the entire process, doing it eight times to the left.

Trunk Twists

Purpose: To tighten waistline and limber upper back.

Stand tall, with your feet about three feet apart. Your arms are stretched out long to the sides at shoulder height. Turn your head to the right and twist your torso as far to the right as you can without having to adjust your feet. Now turn your head to the left and twist your torso to the left. Repeat this entire sequence twenty times.

The Pinwheel

Purpose: To limber torso and tighten waistline.

Stand with your feet about three feet apart. Bend forward from your hips so that your shoulders are in a parallel line with your hips. Your arms are stretched to the sides at shoulder height. Turn your head to the right, your right arm reaching behind you, your left arm reaching in front of you. Now, in the

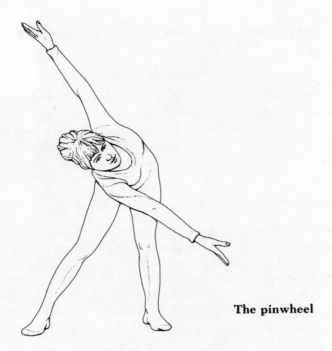

The pinwheel

same manner, turn your head to the left and reverse this pattern. Complete this entire sequence eight times.

ROTATIONAL EXERCISES: "OILING THE JOINTS"

The rotational exercises are specifically designed to realign your hip and pelvic joints. This area has been completely opened due to pregnancy and needs special attention to keep it from either stiffening up or becoming weak and unsupportive of the vital organs the pelvic girdle houses.

The Belly Dancer

Purpose: To increase flexibility in and realign the pelvic joints.

Stand comfortably, with your feet directly under your hips. Bend your knees slightly and place your hands on your hips. Press your pelvis forward and slowly circle your hips to the right, to the back, and finally to the front again. Repeat this sequence eight times to the right and then eight times to the left.

The Figure 8

Purpose: To increase flexibility in and realign the pelvic joints.

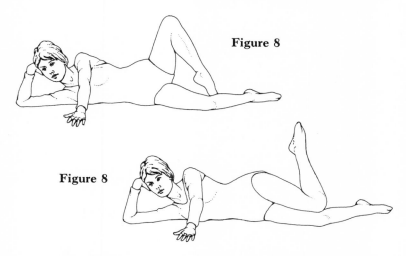

Figure 8

Figure 8

Lie on your back, with both of your knees bent and the soles of your feet touching. Arms are stretched out on the floor on a diagonal, palms facing down. Lift your right knee upward so that it forms a right angle with your torso. Imagine the figure 8 lying on its side in the plane directly in front of you. This 8 should be about four to five feet long. Slowly begin to trace the 8 with the tip of your knee—back and forth, back and forth, until you have completed the 8 about ten times. Now do the same with your left leg.

The Frog

Purpose: To increase flexibility in and realign the pelvic joints.

Kneel and sit down on your heels. Hold your ankles with both of your hands. Slowly, while arching your neck and spine backward, press your pelvis as far forward as possible. Hold the position for a slow count of two. Now slowly reverse this arch and sit back down on your heels. Repeat this exercise four times.

Toe to Knee

Purpose: To increase flexibility in and realign the pelvic joints.

Lie on your left side. Bend your left elbow to support your head, and bend both of your knees slightly. Rotate your right leg in the hip socket so that the front of your right knee is touching the right side of your left leg. The lower portion of your right leg (from the knee down) should be trying to simulate a right angle with the upper portion of your right leg. (This, of course, could never actually happen, unless you are double-jointed.) Now reverse this rotation in your hip and bring your right toe to your left knee with your right knee facing the ceiling. Complete this entire process eight times. Lie on your right side and complete the exercise using your left leg.

Leg Swings

Purpose: To increase flexibility in and realign the pelvic joints.

Stand comfortably and hold onto a doorknob or the back of a chair with your left hand. Bend your right knee slightly and allow it to hang limply from your hip socket. Swing your leg to the front keeping your right knee bent but being careful not to tip the upper body too severely in any direction. Now, using momentum, swing your right leg to the back. Continue this swinging motion for ten sets of forward and backward swings. When you have finished with the right leg, turn around and repeat the exercise using your left leg.

GETTING STRONG: THE STRENGTHENING EXERCISES

The strengthening exercises are designed to tighten your pelvis, buttocks, abdomen, and legs—those areas which have significantly lost their tautness during the months of pregnancy.

YOUR PELVIS AND BUTTOCKS

Your pelvic muscles and buttocks have become loose and toneless due to your pregnancy. Strength in these areas is essential, not merely desirable. Without it, we lose support for our

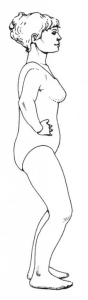
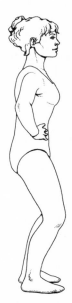

Before exercise program   **After one year of successful exercising**

spine, bowels, bladder, stomach, and reproductive organs. Proper strengthening exercises in these areas can both prevent and remedy countless disturbances such as lower-back pain, incontinence, and even constipation.

The Pelvic Rock

Purpose: To strengthen abdomen, buttocks, and inner thighs; to release tension in the lower back.

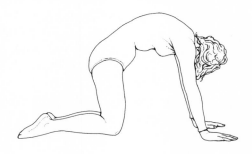

The pelvic rock

Start on your hands and knees. The insides of your legs should be touching. Knees should be in a parallel line to your shoulders. Your spine is straight and parallel to the floor. Look at the floor so that your neck is in line with your spine. Press your stomach down toward the floor. Lift your chin and head and look upward. Your buttocks are tilted toward the ceiling. Elbows are straight. Slowly, begin to curve your spine in the opposite direction while pressing your inner thighs against each other. Now, while pulling your abdominal muscles flat against your lower back, squeeze your buttock muscles tightly together. Look down at your stomach. Your elbows are slightly bent. Hold this position for four counts, keeping the abdominal, the inner-thigh, and the buttock muscles tightly contracted. Repeat this exercise from the beginning eight times.

The Pelvic Tuck

Purpose: To strengthen abdomen, buttocks, inner thighs; to release tension in the lower back.

Lie on the floor or a soft mat with both of your knees bent. Both of your elbows are bent, with your hands relaxed on your chest. Keep both of your feet flat on the floor. Squeeze your buttocks tightly together and press your inner thighs against each other. Contract your abdominal muscles so that your abdomen is flat against your lower back. Lift your pelvis slightly off the floor. Do not arch your lower back. Return to your beginning position. Complete eight times.

The Big Squeeze

Purpose: To strengthen inner thighs and pelvic muscles.

You will need a tennis ball for this exercise. Sit tall on the floor with your spine perfectly straight. If you are more comfortable with a back support, you may sit against the wall. Both knees are bent and your feet are flat on the floor. Place the tennis ball between your knees. Using your inner thigh muscles, press the ball as tightly as possible for four counts. Relax. Complete this exercise six times.

The Silent Squeeze

Purpose: Specifically to strengthen the pelvic muscles.

This exercise can be done virtually in any position—sitting, lying down, standing. Imagine the sensation of having a full bladder and nowhere conveniently to eliminate. Tighten the pelvic muscles, hold two counts, and release. You may perform up to thirty repetitions of this exercise at a time, for there is no strain involved. For a thorough tightening of the pelvic musculature, it is recommended that you complete three sets of thirty repetitions daily.

The Tilt

Purpose: To tighten buttocks and the backs of the legs.

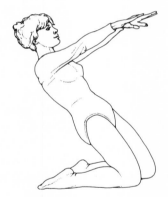

The tilt

Kneel on the floor with both arms extended in front of you for balance. Your knees are in a parallel line with your hips. Keeping your knees, hips, and shoulders in a straight line, tighten your buttocks and tilt your torso backward. Hold for two counts. Return to the beginning position. Repeat this exercise eight times.

The Incline

Purpose: To tighten buttocks and the backs of the legs.

Lie on your stomach on the floor or a soft mat with both

legs stretched out behind you. Your arms are folded to support your head; you can achieve this by bending your elbows and crossing your arms so that your forehead can rest comfortably on your forearms. Squeeze your buttocks while pressing your pelvis down into the floor, and slowly lift both of your legs a few inches off the floor with both your knees straight and your toes pointed. Repeat this exercise eight times.

The Swimmer

Purpose: To tighten buttocks and the backs of the legs.

Start in the same beginning position as you did for "The Incline." Squeeze your buttocks, press your pelvis down into the floor, and lift both your legs with your knees straight and your toes pointed. Hold this position. Kick your legs as you would if you were swimming—that is, one leg lowering as the other rises. Do not allow either leg to touch the floor. Alternate these kicks for six counts and lower both legs. Repeat entire exercise from the beginning. Complete this exercise four times.

The Fish

Purpose: To strengthen the backs of the legs and buttocks.

Start in the same beginning position as you did for "The Incline." Squeeze your buttocks, press your pelvis down into the floor, and lift both of your legs with your knees straight and your toes pointed. Your legs should be about two feet apart when lifted. Breathe in to prepare, and exhale as you bring the insides of your legs together, still keeping both of your legs off the floor. Breathe in, spread your legs apart. Exhale, bring them together. Repeat eight times and then lower both of your legs to the floor.

YOUR ABDOMEN

Whether you have had a natural childbirth or a cesarean section, your abdominal muscles will need specific exercises for you to restore a firm, flat stomach. Because the lower spine has no primary musculature of its own, your stomach muscles are its only real support. Without strong abdominals, locomotor activity (activity which involves moving from one place to another—for example, walking, crawling, running) can become difficult and stressful. The following exercises will create the healthy abdominal support your lower back so vitally needs.

Pullbacks

Purpose: To strengthen your abdominal wall.

Begin seated on the floor or a mat, with both of your knees bent, your feet flat on the floor, and the insides of your legs touching. Fold your arms loosely over your chest, palms above your breastbone. Breathe in and fill your abdomen with air. Exhale and press your abdomen firmly against your lower back. Drop your chin in to your chest, squeeze your buttocks, and press the insides of your legs tightly against each other. Very slowly begin to lower your upper body backwards to the floor. Stop when the tip of your "tailbone" touches the floor. Hold this position for two counts. Breathe in and fill your abdomen with air again. Exhale and pull your abdomen flat against your lower back. Lower your upper body until your waistline touches the floor. Hold this position for two counts. Breathe in and fill your abdomen with air. Exhale, and press your abdomen flat against your lower back. Lower your upper body until your shoulder girdle touches the floor (your head should still be off the floor). Hold this position for two counts. Breathe in one final time. Exhale and slowly lower your head to the floor. This exercise should be completed four times.

Pelvic Sit-ups

Purpose: To strengthen abdominal wall and inner thighs.

Sit erect on the floor or a mat with your shoulders relaxed. Your knees should be bent so that the soles of your feet are touching. Stretch both of your arms directly in front of you at shoulder height. Breathe in and fill your abdomen with air. Exhale, press your abdominal muscles up against your lower back, and drop your chin down in to your chest. Squeeze your

buttocks and slowly begin to roll back to the floor, always keeping your arms at shoulder level. Make sure you lower your
spine one vertebra at a time. When you reach the floor, breathe
in again. Exhale, flatten your abdomen against your lower
back, and bring your chin down into your chest. Now reverse
this entire process and slowly return to the beginning position.
Repeat the complete exercise eight times.

The Twist

Purpose: To strengthen your abdominal wall and tighten waistline.

Lie on your back and draw your knees up in to your chest.
Your arms should be extended level with your shoulders. Now
roll your hips to the right side in an attempt to touch your
knees to the floor. As you are rolling your hips to the right, turn
your head to the left and twist your upper body to the left with
your arms still extended to shoulder level. Pull your stomach
flat against your lower spine and return to the beginning position. Repeat this exercise ten times. Now reverse the entire
exercise, so that you are rolling your hips to the left and twist-
ing your upper body to the right. Repeat this ten times.

The Tummy Press

Purpose: To strengthen abdominal wall, the front of the thighs,
and the backs of the legs.

Lie on your back with both of your knees bent up in to
your chest. Flex both of your feet back as far as they will go
(this action helps to work both sides of your legs simultaneously, rather than just the front). Breathe in to begin. Exhale, flatten your stomach against your lower spine, and straighten both
of your legs, feet still flexed, to form a right angle with your
upper body. At the same time, bring your chin in to your chest,
lift both of your arms off the floor, and reach with your fingertips to touch your toes. (Don't panic if you are not able to touch
your toes immediately. This will come with regular practice.
Just reach as far as you can.) Inhale and return to your begin-

ning position. Repeat this exercise ten times.

The "Pedaling" Tummy Press

Purpose: To strengthen abdominal wall and the front of the thighs.

Lie back on your back with both of your knees in to your chest, keep your feet flexed. Breathe in, press your stomach against your lower back, and straighten your right leg. At the same time, bring your chin in to your chest, lift your upper body, and reach with both arms to your right toe. Inhale and return to the beginning position. Repeat the same procedure, using your left leg. Do this exercise in an alternating action twenty times (ten times with the right leg and ten times with the left).

YOUR LEGS

Your legs have also suffered due to your pregnancy. If you have developed varicose veins, and even if you haven't, proper circulation in the legs becomes essential. Your legs may have developed cellulite, or fatty deposits, especially around the outer sides of the upper thighs (see "The Scourge of Cellulite," Chapter Two). These little fat pockets, often referred to as "maternal stores," may interfere with the function of your musculature, because the fat actually gets trapped in the muscle. Proper exercise, of course, can remedy all of this. The difficulty with leg exercise, which is often overlooked, is that legs have four separate sets of muscles and all of these have to be strengthened separately to obtain the maximum results. The following exercises are designed to work all four sets of leg muscles to restore their former shape and strength.

Leg Lifts

Purpose: To strengthen the front of the thigh.

Lie on your back with your left knee bent and your left foot flat on the floor. Stretch your right leg along the floor. Your arms are relaxed at your sides. Breathe in to begin. Exhale, flatten your stomach up against your lower back, and slowly begin to lift your right leg to form a right angle with your upper body. Keep your leg straight and hold this position for a slow count of two. Again breathe in and exhale, pressing your stomach up against your lower back. Slowly lower your leg and return to the beginning position. Repeat this exercise ten times and then repeat the entire procedure with your left leg.

Inner Thigh Leg Lifts

Purpose: To strengthen the front of the legs and the inner leg muscles.

Follow the same procedure described in "Leg Lifts," with one exception. Keep the leg that is being lifted rotated outward in the hip socket so as to work the inner leg muscles.

The Scissors

Purpose: To strengthen inner leg muscles.

Lie on your back, your arms relaxed at your sides. Both of your legs are extended up, to form a right angle with your upper body. Allow your legs to fall open to the sides so that they form a "V." Breathe in to begin. Exhale, press your stomach up against your lower back, and lift both of your legs, keeping your knees straight, back to the beginning position. Breathe in and open your legs to the sides. Breathe out and close them together. Repeat this exercise ten times.

Outer Thigh Leg Lifts

Purpose: To strengthen outer thighs and calves.

Lie on your left side with both of your knees bent so that the upper portion of your legs (from the knee up) forms a right angle with your upper body. Your left arm is stretched out beyond your head, with the palm down on the floor, to form a pillow for your head. Extend your right leg fully forward, with your right foot flexed to form a right angle with your upper body. Your right toe should be several inches off the ground to begin. Slowly lift your right leg three or four inches and then lower to the beginning position. Repeat twenty times. Reverse entire process and repeat with your left leg extended.

Rotary Leg Lifts

Purpose: To strengthen outer thighs and calves.

Begin in the exact position you did for "Outer Thigh Leg Lifts." Instead of lifting your leg, begin to make a clockwise circular motion, using your entire leg. Complete ten circles. Reverse and complete ten counterclockwise circles. (*Note:* Your leg should not touch the floor until the completion of the exercise.) Now begin this procedure using your left leg. Do ten times each.

Inner Thigh Kicks

Purpose: To strengthen inner thigh.

Lie on your right side with your right leg stretched underneath you. Bend your left knee so that it is perpendicular to your body. Your left knee should be facing the ceiling and the sole of your left foot should be flat on the floor behind your right knee. Your right arm is stretched overhead, palm down on the floor, to cushion your head. Your left arm is resting on the floor in front of your chest in order to support the rest of your body. With your right foot flexed, kick your right leg up off the floor about six to ten inches. Hold this position for a slow count of two and then slowly lower your leg to within an inch of the floor. Repeat this exercise ten times. Then lower your right leg all the way to the floor. Lie on your left side and repeat this procedure with your left leg.

Back Leg Lifts

Purpose: To strengthen the backs of the legs and the buttocks.

Lie on your stomach, your head turned to one side. Your arms are relaxed at your sides. Breathe in to begin and as you exhale, squeeze your buttocks tightly together and lift your right leg four to five inches off the floor. Inhale and lower your right leg to within one inch of the floor. (*Note*: Do bring your leg back to the floor until the completion of this exercise.) Repeat this exercise fifteen times and then lower your right leg all the way to the floor. Now complete the exercise fifteen times with your left leg.

Back Kicks

Purpose: To strengthen the backs of the legs and the buttocks. Kneel on your hands and knees. Bend your knee in to your chest and then slowly extend it all the way to the back. Repeat this fifteen times. Then repeat fifteen times using your left leg.

FOR RELAXATION

There will be times when you are unusually tense or stiff after the completion of an exercise session. This is especially true when you first begin this program. I personally like to conclude any session with the following group of relaxation exercises. They help me unwind and refocus my energy. Also, if you find yourself unable to fall asleep due to a hectic day's schedule, these relaxation exercises may be just the sedative you need.

Constructive rest position

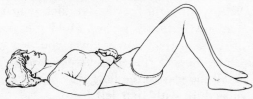

BREATHING EXERCISES (CONTROLLED BREATHING)

Sitting with your legs crossed "Indian style" and your hands relaxed in your lap, inhale through your nose and fill your lungs and diaphragm with air. Now, exhale through your mouth and flatten your abdomen against your lower back. Repeat ten times and rest.

HEAD ROLLS

Begin seated with your legs crossed "Indian style" and your hands relaxed in your lap. Inhale and slowly begin to circle your head to the right, to the back, to the left, and to the front. Make four complete circles. Reverse and circle, beginning to the left, four times.

SHOULDER STRETCHES

Sit with your legs crossed "Indian style" and your hands relaxed in your lap. Slowly begin to circle your shoulders forward, upward, and then to the back. Complete four times and then repeat the entire process, starting to the back.

THE FETAL POSITION

Kneel. Now, keeping your heels directly underneath your buttocks, sit down on your heels. Curl your upper body forward until your forehead reaches your knees. Keep both of your hands gently clasped behind your back. Remain in this position three to five minutes and breathe deeply.

BUTTOCK ROLLS

Lie on your back with your arms stretched to the sides at shoulder level. Both of your knees are bent into you chest. Slowly roll your hips to the right, keeping your shoulder girdle on the floor. Lift your legs back to the beginning position and roll your legs to the left. Repeat this exercise ten times.

Suggested Exercise Sequences/Routines

It is difficult to find agreement in any group of athletes regarding the proper sequence of exercise. Some want to stretch, then strengthen. Others want the reverse. Some want to stretch one day and do strengthening the next. How you go about it really is up to you. However, my personal preference is to warm up first, then stretch, then do strengthening exercises, and finally to wind down with some relaxation exercises. This kind of exercise sequence allows the body gradually to build to a climax and then relax. I find this leaves you the least prone to injury and is best for people who are not experienced in exercise.

The five programs of exercise that I have formulated are organized sequentially. Program I was essentially developed for the first two weeks of postpartum recovery for which you have your doctor's consent to resume exercising. This will generally be from six to twelve weeks after your delivery. Your scheduling for this program should be three one-half-hour periods per week. I recommend that every postpartum mother, regardless of previous physical condition, begin with this program for her own protection. I say this because you are not always aware of just how much your body has changed due to pregnancy. You may take on an activity you think you are familiar with but in reality are not, and may suffer a strained muscle as a result. Do the exercises in Program I exactly as they are planned in sequence, in schedule, and in the number of repetitions. If you are in particularly good shape and honestly feel that Program I is not strenuous enough for you, you may advance to Program II after your first week of exercise.

Program II encompasses the second two weeks of your exercise program. Its schedule requires three forty-minute periods per week. Repetitions of various exercises will increase and new exercises will be included. If you are wondering why I include more of one kind of exercise than another—say, more pelvic than abdominal exercises in the beginning—it is because certain body parts heal more slowly than others and must not be strained initially.

Program III, IV, and V follow the same kind of formula. Program III is the two-month program, Program IV is the three-month program, and Program V is for six months. As your level of proficiency increases, so do the difficulty, the scheduling, and the repetitions of a given exercise.

You may not be able to do every single exercise each session, no matter how efficient you become. However, it is true that as you become more capable, it will take you less time to perform a given set of exercises. If this were not true, your schedule would become a three-hour period rather than a one-hour period. The more difficult the program, the more strenuous the exercise itself and the number of repetitions I suggest. To compensate for this in the later programs, I have eliminated some of the earlier exercises which served to prepare your body for the more strenuous ones.

Program V is actually a maintenance program. If you exercise consistently for the year following your child's birth, you will notice a significant change in your body. Hopefully, it will be better than it ever was. And you will want to maintain this "new you" for a lifetime.

I include two numbers in my repetition column in Program V. The first is your basic schedule repeat number—the number of times you do an exercise in your regular three-times-weekly program. The second is your maximum number. This number is a kind of "check-up" system. Once every six weeks (after the first year of exercise) do an hourly session performing all of your exercises at maximum level. This will be a test to see what "really good shape" you are in!

PROGRAM I: TWO WEEKS
Schedule: Three half-hour periods per week

STRETCHING YOUR BODY	REPETITIONS
WARMING UP	
Chin to Knee	4× each leg
The Lunge	1× each leg
Arm Crosses	5×
Knee Pulls	4× each leg
Side Bends	4× each side

Stretching Your Body (cont.)	Repetitions
YOUR PELVIS	
The Pelvic Stretch	1×
YOUR BACK	
The Cobra	1×
YOUR LEGS	
The "V"	2×
YOUR TORSO AND WAISTLINE	
Standing Side Stretch	4× each side
Trunk Twists	8×

Rotational Exercises

The Belly Dancer	4× each side
The Figure 8	4× each side

Getting Strong: The Strengthening Exercises

YOUR PELVIS AND BUTTOCKS	
The Pelvic Rock	4×
The Pelvic Tuck	4×
The Big Squeeze	2×
The Silent Squeeze	3 sets of 30 repetitions *daily*
YOUR LEGS	
Leg Lifts	5× each leg

For Relaxation

Breathing Exercises	10×
Head Rolls	4× each side
Shoulder Stretches	4× each direction
The Fetal Position	one complete time
Buttock Rolls	10×

PROGRAM II: TWO WEEKS
Schedule: Three forty-minute periods per week

STRETCHING YOUR BODY	REPETITIONS
WARMING UP	
Chin to Knee	4× each leg
The Lunge	1× each leg
Arm Crosses	10×
Knee Pulls	4× each leg
Side Bends	4× each side
YOUR PELVIS	
The Pelvic Stretch	2×
The Pelvic Floor Stretch	4× each side
YOUR BACK	
The Cobra	2×
YOUR LEGS	
The "V"	2×
Wall Stretching	2×
Long Leg Stretch	4× each leg
YOUR TORSO AND WAISTLINE	
Standing Side Stretch	4× each side
Trunk Twists	8×
The Pinwheel	4×

ROTATIONAL EXERCISES: "OILING THE JOINTS"

The Frog	2×
Toe to Knee	4× each leg
Leg Swings	5× each leg

GETTING STRONG:
THE STRENGTHENING EXERCISES   REPETITIONS

YOUR PELVIS AND BUTTOCKS

The Big Squeeze   4×
The Silent Squeeze   3 sets of 30 repetitions
                                     daily

The Tilt   4×
The Incline   4×

YOUR ABDOMEN

Pullbacks   1×

FOR RELAXATION

Breathing Exercises   10×
Head Rolls   4× each side
Shoulder Stretches   4× each direction
The Fetal Position   one complete time
Buttock Rolls   10×

PROGRAM III: TWO MONTHS
Schedule: Four half-hour periods per week

STRETCHING YOUR BODY   REPETITIONS

WARMING UP

Chin to Knee   4× each leg
The Lunge   1× each leg
Arm Crosses   10×
Knee Pulls   4× each leg
Side Bends   4× each side

STRETCHING YOUR BODY (*cont.*)	REPETITIONS
YOUR PELVIS	
The Pelvic Floor Stretch	4× each side
The Wide Pelvic Floor Stretch	4×
YOUR BACK	
The Bow	1×
The Plow	1×
The Forward Bend	4×
The Triangle	1×
YOUR LEGS	
The "V"	2×
Wall Stretching	2×
Long Leg Stretch	4× each leg
YOUR TORSO AND WAISTLINE	
Standing Side Stretch	4× each side
Trunk Twists	10×
The Pinwheel	4×

ROTATIONAL EXERCISES: "OILING THE JOINTS"

The Frog	2×
Toe to Knee	8× each leg
Leg Swings	10× each leg

GETTING STRONG: THE STRENGTHENING EXERCISES

YOUR PELVIS AND BUTTOCKS	
The Big Squeeze	6×
The Silent Squeeze	3 sets of 30 repetitions *daily*
The Tilt	4×
The Incline	4×

GETTING STRONG *(cont.)*	REPETITIONS
YOUR ABDOMEN	
Pullbacks	2×
Pelvic Sit-ups	4×
YOUR LEGS	
Leg Lifts	5× each leg
Inner Thigh Leg Lifts	4× each leg
The Scissors	5×
Outer Thigh Leg Lifts	10× each leg

FOR RELAXATION

Breathing Exercises	10×
Head Rolls	4× each side
Shoulder Stretches	4× each direction
The Fetal Position	one complete time
Buttock Rolls	10×

PROGRAM IV: THREE MONTHS
Schedule: Four half-hour periods per week

STRETCHING YOUR BODY	REPETITIONS
WARMING UP	
Chin to Knee	4× each leg
The Lunge	1× each leg
Arm Crosses	10×
Knee Pulls	4× each leg
Side Bends	4× each side
YOUR PELVIS	
The Pelvic Floor Stretch	8× each side
The Wide Pelvic Floor Stretch	8×

STRETCHING YOUR BODY (*cont.*)   REPETITIONS

YOUR BACK

The Bow	4×
The Plow	2×
The Forward Bend	8×
The Triangle	one complete time

YOUR LEGS

Wall Stretching	2×
Long Leg Stretch	8× each leg

YOUR TORSO AND WAISTLINE

Trunk Twists	20×
The Pinwheel	8×

ROTATIONAL EXERCISES: "OILING THE JOINTS"

The Frog	4×
Leg Swings	10× each leg

GETTING STRONG: THE STRENGTHENING EXERCISES

YOUR PELVIS AND BUTTOCKS

The Big Squeeze	6×
The Silent Squeeze	3 sets of 30 repetitions *daily*
The Tilt	8×
The Incline	8×
The Swimmer	2×
The Fish	2×

YOUR ABDOMEN

The Twist	5× each side
The Tummy Press	5×
The "Pedaling" Tummy Press	5× each leg

GETTING STRONG (*cont.*)   REPETITIONS

YOUR LEGS

Inner Thigh Leg Lifts	10× each leg
The Scissors	10×
Outer Thigh Leg Lifts	10× each leg
Rotary Leg Lifts	5× in each direction with each leg
Inner Thigh Kicks	5× each leg
Back Leg Lifts	10× each leg
Back Kicks	10× each leg

FOR RELAXATION

Breathing Exercises	10×
Head Rolls	4× each side
Shoulder Stretches	4× each direction
The Fetal Position	one complete time
Buttock Rolls	10×

PROGRAM V: MAINTENANCE
Schedule: Three one-hour periods per week

STRETCHING YOUR BODY   REPETITIONS

WARMING UP

Chin to Knee	4× each leg
The Lunge	1× each leg
Arm Crosses	10×
Knee Pulls	4× each leg
Side Bends	8× each side

YOUR PELVIS

The Pelvic Floor Stretch	8× (10× max.) each side

STRETCHING YOUR BODY (cont.)	REPETITIONS
The Wide Pelvic Floor Stretch	8× (10× max.) each side

YOUR BACK

The Bow	4× (6× max.)
The Plow	2× (6× max.)
The Forward Bend	8× (10× max.)
The Triangle	one complete time

YOUR LEGS

Wall Stretching	2× (6× max.)
Long Leg Stretch	8× (10× max.) each leg

ROTATIONAL EXERCISES: "OILING THE JOINTS"

The Frog	4× (6× max.)
Leg Swings	10× (15× max.)

GETTING STRONG: THE STRENGTHENING EXERCISES

YOUR PELVIS AND BUTTOCKS

The Big Squeeze	6× (8× max.)
The Silent Squeeze	3 sets of 30 repetitions *daily*
The Tilt	8× (10× max.)
The Incline	8× (10× max.)
The Swimmer	4× (6× max.)
The Fish	4× (6× max.)

YOUR ABDOMEN

The Twist	10× (12× max.) each side
The Tummy Press	10× (12× max.)

Getting Strong (cont.)	Repetitions
The "Pedaling" Tummy Press	10× (12× max.) each leg

YOUR LEGS

Inner Thigh Leg Lifts	10× (12× max.) each leg
The Scissors	10× (12× max.)
Outer Thigh Leg Lifts	20× (25× max.) each leg
Rotary Leg Lifts	10× (12× max.) in each direction with each leg
Inner Thigh Kicks	10× (12× max.) each leg
Back Leg Kicks	15× (20× max.) each leg
Back Kicks	15× (20× max.) each leg

FOR RELAXATION

Breathing Exercises	10×
Head Rolls	4× each side
Shoulder Stretches	4× each direction
The Fetal Position	one complete time
Buttock Rolls	10×

If you have never before persevered in a regular exercise program, and even if you have, the previous exercises offer a unique opportunity for you to begin a lifetime of fitness. Exercise can improve your appearance, your strength, your health, and your mental attitude. You deserve to be in top physical condition both for yourself and for those who love you and depend upon you.

=4=

Breast-feeding: Pro and Con

During the past ten years, due to the pioneering work of such support groups as the La Leche League, almost 50 percent of all American mothers have nursed their newborn babies—compared to less than 25 percent who made the choice to breast-feed their infants twenty-five years ago. Breast milk is the cleanest, safest, and purest food for your baby. It is accessible, is always the right temperature, and is in a constant supply for most healthy women. Most pediatricians now recommend that you nurse your baby for at least a short time. There is virtually nothing undesirable about the philosophy of breast-feeding, which promotes the use of the substantially nutritious breast milk and the intimacy which a mother develops by nursing her infant.

The La Leche League was founded in 1956 by several mothers as a result of their own need for nursing information. The La Leche League has now expanded to over 3000 individual groups in the United States, with branches in forty-three foreign countries. Each group holds discussion meetings on topics related to nursing and has information on breast-feeding, on a telephone "hotline" manned by mothers nursing their children and by medical consultants, available to all mothers who are nursing their infants. The La Leche League philosophy is to promote successful breast-feeding for all healthy new mothers.

However, in their zealousness to promote the many benefits of nursing, I believe that some supporters of breast-feeding have done the contemporary woman a disservice. Breast-feeding should be presented as a choice—a very good choice, but a choice nonetheless. There is actually some literature about breast-feeding that accuses the mother who is not breast-feeding her child of being neurotic or frigid. "A truly maternal mother," one pamphlet states, should be "grief-stricken at the thought of weaning." I strongly feel that this kind of material does more harm than good and that the concept of being grief-stricken at the termination of nursing is actually more neurotic than choosing not to nurse a child.

The woman who chooses not to nurse her baby is just as concerned and loving a mother as the one who chooses to do so. Some literature on breast-feeding promotes the notion that mothers who do not breast-feed their children may abuse them simply because they have chosen not to do so. There are absolutely no viable data to confirm this theory. A woman who is abusing her children has deeply rooted emotional conflicts that developed long before she made a decision whether or not to nurse her child.

It is my opinion, and the opinion of experts and pediatricians, that a new mother should begin to nurse her child only when she truly wants to and continue only as long as she wants. It is true that some women, who are ignorant of the nature of breast-feeding, may reject it simply due to lack of proper information. However, there are many women who have been adequately educated and still may choose against breast-feeding for a variety of legitimate reasons.

I had a very demanding job and economically I couldn't afford to stay home. I never was able to relax enough or find adequate time to breast-feed my child successfully.

I started breast-feeding my baby but I couldn't continue. I didn't fit into my clothes properly. I just didn't feel comfortable about myself.

Breast-feeding—no. I didn't even consider it. The bottle is a perfectly wonderful invention.

However, many mothers not nursing their children continue to feel guilty about their choice to bottle-feed them. And there is really no need to feel this way. An ill-nourished or cigarette-smoking mother who is breast-feeding her child can never hope to compete with an adequately made formula. It is interesting that women who have had cesarean deliveries rather than vaginal deliveries experience the same guilty feeling— about resorting to an alternative method of birthing—as do mothers who have chosen not to breast-feed their babies. The assumption is that you are more of a woman if you birth your children naturally and feed them naturally than if you use the available alternatives. The beliefs, however, are biased and may be responsible for lowering a woman's self-esteem at a time when she needs self-confidence and support. No woman should feel guilty about her choice of feeding method. I have listed the advantages and disadvantages of both in the chart on the following page.

If you do choose to breast-feed your baby, take heed that it is not going to be easy. Breast-feeding is a learned response. It takes practice and commitment. (See also "How to Nurse Your Child" in this chapter.) If you can persevere through the initial discomfort, you can discover a wonderful experience in intimacy.

If you choose to bottle-feed your child or supplement breast-feeding with formula, I strongly suggest that you make your own. Some commercial brands of formula are laced with sugar, corn syrup, or other sugar derivatives. Sugar can be detrimental to your baby and should be avoided. Some health-food stores sell soya-based (soybean-derivative) formula and

Breast	*Bottle*
PRO Milk is readily available at the proper temperature. No need for sterilization.	*CON* Milk needs preparation. Milk needs to be heated. Bottles may need to be sterilized. (*Note:* There is research to indicate that sterilization may be an unnecessary practice, but as yet, this is not confirmed.)
PRO Milk is economical.	*CON* Formula components must be purchased and thus incur some expense.
PRO Milk contains vital antibodies that protect your baby against infection.	*CON* No substitute is available.
CON Mother cannot tell exactly how much milk has been ingested without weighing her baby.	*PRO* Mother can tell immediately how much milk her baby has taken.
CON Mother's basic health and diet directly affect the quality of the milk.	*PRO* Milk quality is independent of mother's health.
CON Milk supply normally but not *always* adjusts itself to the needs of the baby.	*PRO* Extra feedings are available upon demand.
CON Drugs and other medication filter into the milk.	*PRO* Mother's medication cannot affect her baby.

powdered goat's milk. Both of these products are fairly close in composition to mother's milk and are thus satisfactory substitutes. Again, always remember to check with your pediatrician before you begin to feed any formula to your baby.

I find the following formula, first promoted by Adelle Davis, the best substitute or supplement for breast milk. This formula can be made directly in the bottle:

Formula:

   3 ounces evaporated milk, or soy milk if milk allergy has been diagnosed
   4½ ounces water
   2 teaspoons either lactose (milk sugar) or maltose dextrin mixture (combination of grain and grape sugar available in health-food stores)
   1 teaspoon liquid acidophilus culture, available at health-food stores. (*Note:* Acidophilus culture is an antibody found in yogurt and certain types of milk.)

Pour all these ingredients into your bottle, close it, and shake for ten seconds (all ingredients should be at room temperature). This formula can also be prepared in larger quantities in your blender. Any unused formula can be refrigerated and then heated to room temperature before the next feeding.

You must understand that your initial choice to breast- or bottle-feed your child is not a permanent one. If you begin to nurse him and find yourself unable to continue, you can always switch to bottle-feeding. Surprisingly, even if you begin with bottle-feeding and your milk supply dries up, by using the proper procedure (see "How to Nurse Your Child" in this chapter) you can begin to breast-feed your baby even six months after delivery. This is often done if the infant is found to have allergies to all prepared formulas. There is also no reason to use one of the methods exclusively. Many women, including myself, find that a balanced combination of breast- and bottle-feeding ensures both the intimacy of the breast and the freedom and convenience of the bottle.

Also, when you do make your choice, whatever it may be,

expect someone to disagree with you. Your mother, relatives, and friends may raise an eyebrow when you choose to breast-feed your child. Friends who are breast-feeding their children may gasp as you remove a glass bottle from your purse. The most important point to remember is that you are feeding your baby, not theirs. You don't owe anyone an explanation.

One final note to mothers not breast-feeding their children, since I am going to concentrate on mothers who do for the rest of this chapter, is this: Don't force yourself to nurse your child simply because you feel guilty. If you would like to try for a little while, do so. If it truly disturbs you, then stop. I have known a great many women who resented the act of nursing but continued because they felt society expected it of them. (A similar situation occurred in the reverse during the forties, when all mothers were encouraged to bottle-feed their babies.) They were not the happiest of women, having been pressured into performing an act that was both uncomfortable and perhaps distasteful to them (see also Body Image and Your Breasts, page 166). True, there is a difference in quality between breast milk and formula, but the difference is a mild one—certainly nothing to warrant undue distress. An ambivalent feeling about breast-feeding tends to destroy the very relationship which breast-feeding is supposed to create. Hold your baby close and cuddle him as you bottle feed him. Make eye contact, sing, do anything that pleases you. In this way, you can create a loving, warm relationship with your baby no matter what feeding method you choose.

In the remaining sections in this chapter, I will discuss the anatomy, the mechanics, and the emotional response of the mother breast-feeding her child.

ANATOMY OF A NURTURER

The adult female breast is designed rather like an orange. Each of the fifteen to twenty-five lobes, or segments, of this "orange" has treelike veins embedded in fat and separated by fibrous tissue. Within seventy-two hours after childbirth, milk is produced in the alveoli, the leaflike formations in the lobes, and flows down the smaller ducts into the main duct, or "trunk." Here a reservoir of milky fluid is formed just underneath the areola, the dark area encircling the nipple. Each of the fifteen to twenty-five lobes has a small opening on the nipple.

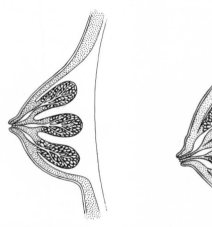

Nonlactating breast   Lactating breast

Milk secretion can begin, and often does, before childbirth, in the last trimester of pregnancy. It is then that the production of the hormones estrogen and progesterone slowly begin to diminish. As these hormone levels taper off, they stimulate the hypothalamus, which in turn causes the pituitary gland to secrete prolactin—the milk-producing hormone. The initial secretions (see also Chapter Two) are not true milk but a yellowish substance known as colostrum. Colostrum is rich in antibodies that are never present in any formula and create an immunity against infection and disease in newborns for up to six months after birth.

The actual milk yield (which begins after seventy-two hours following childbirth) is triggered by the baby's sucking.

This sucking action relays nerve impulses to the hypothalamus, which in turn releases the hormone oxytocin. This hormone (which also causes the uterus to contract after delivery) causes the alveoli to contract and push milk through the ducts and into the nipples. Milk flow will normally begin thirty seconds after sucking commences.

Milk supply can be irregular, especially during the first six weeks of the postpartum period. The most widely spread symptoms of a fluctuating milk supply is milk tension, or engorgement. Since the prolactin level is so high (higher than it will ever be) immediately after childbirth, the breasts of many mothers nursing their children will overfill with milk to the point of discomfort. *Note*: Small-breasted women are particularly susceptible to this condition.) This tension in the breasts inhibits milk secretion. Thus, even if the new mother wishes to nurse her child, milk secretion, or the "let-down reflex," as it is often termed (see also "How to Nurse Your Child" in this chapter) will be slow or even cease temporarily. If your baby is hungry, you can try to nurse him to relieve this tension. If this is not enough, pumping or manual expression (see also "How to Nurse Your Child" in this chapter) every two to three hours can help relieve engorgement. If you are still in pain, wrap a few ice cubes in a soft towel and place over your breasts for ten minutes. The cold will numb the breasts temporarily, ease the pain, and allow you to nurse your child again. Fortunately, the storage capacity of the breast will improve over the next couple of weeks and this problem will cease to exist.

It is not generally known why the breast, after it has been sufficiently "indoctrinated," will almost always produce milk in the right amount. (*Note*: It takes about six weeks to create a good let-down, or secretion, reflex.) If your baby is a "big eater," your breasts will almost always meet his demands. If your baby is a skimpy eater, your breasts will produce only what is needed in a single feeding. What hormones are involved in this highly laudable supply-and-demand reflex are unknown. The conjecture is that somatotropin, the growth hormone involved in breast development, may play a role in milk supply; the thyroid gland, too may be involved. Now let's take a look at the mechanics of the nursing process.

How to Nurse Your Child

Nursing is a very personal experience, and there are as many nursing methods as there are mothers nursing their children. I have chosen to present a variety of alternatives here, so feel free to choose among them.

If you have made the decision to breast-feed your child, take two to three nursing bras to the hospital. You will generally need a cup a size larger than you wore during your pregnancy, so take that into consideration when making your purchase. If you wore well-fitting bras during your pregnancy, your breasts should be relatively firm after delivery. Nursing bras should have a Velcro pad or snap on both straps that can be opened easily but remain secure when closed. This feature enables you to lower each cup portion individually to feed your baby. The most practical bras are made of cotton, to ensure proper ventilation. There should not be a great deal of elastic in the bra, as frequent washing (nursing bras are always wet with milk and thus need to be washed constantly) can stretch elasticized bras out of shape. Most good nursing bras resemble something you may have seen your grandmother wearing. There are more attractive bras available at the more elite department stores, but some of these bras have drawbacks, such as being difficult to undo when you are ready to nurse your child or being uncomfortable to wear. There are, of course, some both adequate and smartly designed bras available, but if you don't know what you are looking for, you may make an inappropriate purchase. Nursing bras are available at both lingerie and maternity shops.

It is also practical to invest in some serviceable nursing clothing. You will be more buxom than usual and your regular clothing may not fit you properly. Since you cannot get completely undressed every time you wish to nurse your baby, it is advisable to purchase clothing that is suitable for nursing. Blouses and sweaters that button down the front are good. So are big, roomy tops that can be discreetly lifted up from the waist. In this way, your baby can gain access to your breasts from underneath and you can fold the rest of your blouse over your breasts and midriff. This is particularly desirable when you are out in public and do not wish to be conspicuous. Dresses, unless they have been specially designed, are not practical. In my particular circumstance, I found leotards effective, I simply wore a tank or short-sleeved leotard and slipped the strap off one shoulder when I wanted to nurse my daughter.

Initially, you will need to purchase breast pads from your drug store. They will absorb any excess milk that may leak and drip onto your clothing. These small, circular pads are made of cotton and are slipped into the cup of your bra. Later on, when your letdown reflex has been fully developed, you will not need them. Many women, however, continue to wear breast pads for the duration of nursing their children just as an added insurance against leakage.

If you are in a hospital where "rooming in" (the baby is kept in the same room as the mother and placed in the nursery only for routine testing or if the mother wants rest) is practiced, you may nurse your baby as soon as he is brought to you. Your baby will be very tired for about forty-eight hours after delivery and will generally have little interest in eating. However, even the smallest amount of colostrum he ingests is good for him at this early time.

You may nurse your baby in a variety of positions, either sitting or lying down. If you are sitting, you can cradle your baby in your right arm, using your left hand to guide your nipple into his mouth—or in reverse, if you are left-handed. A two- or three-day-old infant may be hungry and suck extraordinarily hard, taking most of the areola as well as the nipple into his mouth. Nurse him for five minutes on the right breast and then reverse the process so that you can nurse him five

Nursing positions

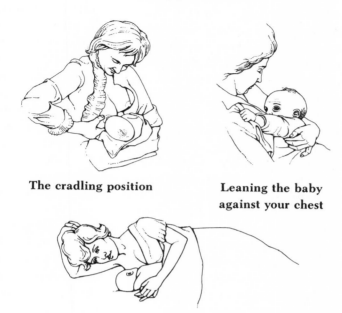

The cradling position   **Leaning the baby
                                   against your chest**

Nursing your baby lying down

minutes on the left breast. Eventually, you can increase your nursing time to fifteen minutes on each breast. There are some doctors who feel that you should nurse your baby from only one breast at each feeding, but most agree that nursing from both breasts will keep one nipple from becoming overly sore at a single feeding. To remove your baby from the breast, simply insert your finger into the side of his mouth to stop the suction. If you don't, he may actually suck harder to remain on the breast.

If you began nursing him on your right breast, begin on your left breast at the subsequent feeding. You can pin a safety pin to your bra to remember which breast to begin nursing him with. (This may sound complicated, but you will become ac-customed to it.) One reason to alternate breasts in this fashion is to produce an equal milk supply in each breast, thereby preventing engorgement or a scanty supply in either breast. By the fourth or fifth day after delivery, your baby will be nursing eight to nine times a day for a half-hour period each time. He may consume anywhere from three to eight ounces of fluid every two to three hours. Your baby will not know day or night for the first three weeks, so he may be more demanding at 4 A.M. than at 2 P.M., for example. This "heavy" feeding schedule will taper off to about six feedings by the third month. Remember, these are only approximations. Some nursing babies eat as often as ten times a day and some as few as five. Some will eat only once during the night or not at all, and others will demand four nightly feedings. The simplest way to avoid the real exhaustion that naturally follows "all-night" feedings is to take the baby to bed with you. Don't believe what your grandmother told you—you will not roll over on your baby and suffocate him; you will never be able to fall into a deep enough sleep for that. Lie on your side with both of your breasts exposed and your baby facing you. In this manner, your baby can gain access to your milk without your having to get out of bed. If your baby can reach only one breast in this position, roll onto the other side holding your baby on your chest. Another method of increasing your sleeping hours is to give your baby two big "meals" before he goes to sleep. One meal could be at 8 P.M. and the other at 11 P.M. This way your baby may be full for four to five hours and allow you to sleep. There is one problem with this method; it doesn't stop milk leakage during the night. After all, your body doesn't know that your baby isn't hungry. You may wake up with a wet chest and soaking sheets. However, it may be to your advantage to be a little wet and get well rested. Besides, this leakage will not continue. Once your let-down reflex has been firmly established, leakage will practically disappear.

A biological explanation of the let-down reflex is simply this. If all the alveoli in the lobes contract during nursing, then all the milk being specifically produced for *your* baby, as a result of the amount of sucking your baby does, is being secreted, or let down. Without a complete let-down reflex, your baby will be able to remove only about one-third of the milk being produced. The rest of the milk will remain in the breast until the next feeding, when it is pushed into the nipples. Without an adequate let-down reflex, your baby will almost always be hungry, since he will not be receiving the last portion of the breast milk, which is generally very rich in fat.

As I have said earlier, nursing is a learned response. It takes about two to three weeks to learn to nurse a child and about two months to acquire a good let-down reflex. As I've indicated, the let-down reflex is simply nature's way of learning how much milk to make. Let's face it, your baby doesn't know whether you've had twins or even triplets. However, once a good let-down reflex is established, your baby will not have to suck as hard or as long for his nourishment, and you will not have to give as many feedings. Your milk will literally pour from your breasts without the initial discomfort you once experienced. There are a few signs that your let-down reflex is beginning to work. As you nurse your baby from one breast, milk will begin to drip from the other. Your nipples will begin to tingle right before you nurse the baby. It is as if your body knows that your baby is ready to eat. Later, your breasts will have a "pins-and-needles" sensation that will be relieved by nursing him.

If you are having trouble with your let-down reflex even after two or three months of nursing your child, your doctor may prescribe a nasal spray containing oxytocin, the let-down hormone. A contributor to the lack of a good let-down reflex can be stress. Of course, you cannot avoid all stress, but you and your family can greatly reduce it. Try to get as much rest as possible.

It is important to understand that no matter how effective your let-down reflex may be, there are going to be days when your baby never seems to get enough to eat and others when he doesn't seem to eat at all. Remember, babies are people too.

They are more hungry at certain times than at others.

The truly amazing fact about nursing a child is that almost any woman can do it. This includes the mothers of adopted babies and even women who have never been pregnant. If a woman has given birth to one child but is unable biologically to have a second one, she can nurse her adopted baby through a process known as relactation. Lact-aid, an amazing device developed by the father of an adopted baby, has been used effectively to stimulate milk production in women who haven't been pregnant for as many as six years. Lact-aid consists of a formula sac with a tube laid alongside the breast. In this manner, the baby does not get frustrated sucking on an empty breast and yet the sucking action is eventually able to create a normal milk supply. Unfortunately, women who have never been pregnant have not been able to establish a full milk supply but have been able to develop a modest amount, which can be supplemented with formula.

As personal as your decision to nurse your child is your decision to wean him. After six months, your baby will be introduced to solid foods and other fluids. The actual physical need for breast milk will cease at this point. If your baby does continue to nurse, because he will be eating other foods he will not be nursing as often. Your milk supply will adapt to this new feeding situation. You may even be able to get a full night's sleep, although some babies will have you up at night well into their first year.

At about the age of nine months, your baby will demonstrate a notable lack of interest in the breast. He may even wish to drink from a cup instead. However, some babies, if encouraged, will go on nursing well into their second year, although they will be nursing only once or twice a day.

The most important thing about weaning is to do it gradually. Don't force the issue. If your baby enjoys juices and solid foods, he may wean himself at six or seven months. As I have said earlier, gradual weaning is better for both you and your baby. Your breasts and your baby's eating patterns will adapt to weaning, as they did to nursing.

Nursing Complications

Mastitis, a common breast infection, often occurs during the initial weeks of nursing. Essentially, what happens is this: Your milk flow is incomplete, and the remaining milk gets plugged or caked in one of your breast ducts. This area becomes red or sensitive to the touch. The first signs of mastitis are fever and an overall sick feeling.

If this happens, call your doctor. Do not stop nursing your baby on the infected breast. Not nursing him will only aggravate your condition, causing the milk flow to back up farther. Your doctor will probably prescribe an antibiotic called Dosycycline. This antibiotic has been developed to have no undesirable effects on your baby.

Place a hot compress (a towel soaked in hot water) on the infected breast for about five minutes once an hour. Continue to nurse your baby on the infected breast or pump it if your baby refuses to eat (see also "How to Nurse Your Child" in this chapter). The sooner you get your milk flowing normally the better.

Breast abscessing, as a result of mastitis, is the collecting of pus in the breast where dead cell tissue has accumulated and not been expelled from the body due to poor circulation. This condition, however, is usually due to infrequent nursing and not to continual nursing on the infected breast.

The causes of early postpartum mastitis are varied, but they include emotional tension and lack of sleep. I personally believe, and am supported by many gynecologists, that one of the major contributors to mastitis is poor circulation, caused by lack of proper exercise. Some doctors and advocates of breast-feeding encourage the new mother to stay in bed a week or more during the initial lactation period, in the belief that inactivity causes you to relax and thus promotes milk secretion. I disagree. Inactivity causes tension and weakened muscles (especially the vital pelvic muscles that need specific attention during this period) and it slows down circulation. Read, sew, do your pelvic exercises, play the piano, but do not sit in bed. I, for

one, was considerably active during the early postpartum period and never had a single breast infection or the same difficulty relaxing as some of my sedentary friends.

At about the twentieth feeding, your nipples may become
irritated and sore due to the sucking action of your baby. They
may even crack or bleed. If this happens and you have enough
privacy in your home, try to expose your nipples to the air and
even the sun. Keep them clean and dry between feedings. Do
not rub your nipples with Vaseline, soap, or alcohol, as is often
suggested. These products will only aggravate your condition.
Although some doctors are totally against the use of plastic
nipple shields, I and a number of gynecologists advocate them,
especially in instances of cracked nipples and nipple soreness. It
is true that the nipple shield, which is simply a rubber nipple
attached to a suction device, will not create enough suction to
empty the breast completely. This inadequate emptying of the
breast may signal your body to produce milk in a smaller
amount at the subsequent feeding (remember the supply-and-
demand reflex), and can result in the baby receiving a relatively small amount of breast milk while your nipples are sore.
I, however, prefer supplying a smaller amount of breast milk
and perhaps supplementing it with formula to not being able to
breast-feed a baby at all because my nipples are so irritated. It
is not always easy to "grin and bear it," as many doctors will
recommend. The nipple shield can get you over "the hump"
before the bleeding begins and allow you to return to normal
feeding when your nipples are no longer sore and irritated.
Also, if your nipples begin to bleed, the sight of blood in your
baby's mouth can make you uneasy. Of course, many doctors
are against this practice because of the temporary fluctuation
in milk supply it creates. These doctors will insist that your
baby suck directly on the breast no matter what. Ultimately,
the decision belongs to you. As long as you don't use a sore
nipple as your sole excuse for discontinuing breast-feeding, I
feel that any method which ensures the continuance of comfortable breast-feeding is one to be considered.

Many women have retracted or inverted nipples, nipples which remain buried in the areola. This condition can make nursing almost unbearable. I have inverted nipples, and I know how uncomfortable this can be. Though some gynecologists recommend the manual pulling and rotating of the nipples with the fingers in order to expose them, research has indicated that this does little good. Other doctors recommend further sex play in the breast area. The sex play, however, is not more comfortable than the nursing, and because it is so painful it is rarely continued. The most effective method of coping with inverted nipples is to use the Woolrich breast shield. Dr. Harold Woller, a British obstetrician, developed this shield, which can be purchased from the La Leche League. These plastic shields are worn inside your bra. They create a gentle suction on the nipples and exert pressure on the areolae. If worn for several weeks, they can virtually eliminate inversion.

If you happen to get sick (catch the flu, a stomach virus, or a bad cold), get yourself to the doctor. Your milk supply, of course, will be lowered due to infection, but you can still nurse your baby. Breast milk contains lysozyme, an enzyme that dissolves bacteria and thus prevents the spread of infection to your baby. So even though your nursing will not protect you from sickness, your baby will be protected. Even breast-fed infants from areas where disease and infection are rampant seem to remain relatively healthy.

Weaning also produces changes in the breasts. During the 1920s it was suggested that weaning be done abruptly. Breasts were bound and fluid intake was restricted. This kind of weaning (see also "How to Nurse Your Child" in this chapter) is nothing short of disastrous to the mother. Abrupt weaning causes the breasts first to become engorged with milk (which often causes extreme pain) and then to become empty within several days. The best method is to allow the child to wean himself slowly and naturally. If the weaning is gradual, there will be no pain or discomfort and the breasts will return to their prepregnant state in about six months.

"I HAVE NO FREEDOM." BEING TIED DOWN

The best statement about the emotional condition of the mother breast-feeding her child came from one of my exercise students. She sat comfortably in our carpeted vestibule, suckling her baby. Another woman, who was discussing her career, turned to the mother and asked what she did, meaning of course, her profession. The new mother turned to her and said: "Well, I used to teach remedial reading. Now, I breast-feed my baby."

Breast-feeding, if unsupplemented, can become a full-time career. It can seem as if you and your baby either sleep or are in the process of feeding. Before your baby can ingest solid foods, which usually begins on or about his six-month birthday, your milk is his only source of nourishment. His hunger can, at times, be overpowering emotionally as well as physically. You cannot go anywhere alone, even if you hire a baby-sitter, unless you can be home in two hours for a feeding.

Although there are many promoters of breast-feeding who frown on the use of the bottle outside an absolute emergency, I feel that its implementation can save many a mother from resentment and frustration. If you don't wish to use formula, you must learn to express your milk and store it for future use. This way, you can leave your breast milk with your husband, relative, or baby-sitter and you can have a well-deserved outing. The first method I wish to discuss is manual expression, or expression by hand. Manual expression is easier for some women than it is for others. Some women actually prefer it to expressing with a device. It is best to express manually when your breast is not too full. If you try to express milk from a full breast, it may be uncomfortable to do. Squeeze the areola behind your nipple between your thumb and your index finger or press your areola up against the side of a glass. At first your milk will come in drops and then in a fine spray. Perform this procedure for both of your breasts. The more you express your milk, the greater amounts of milk will be released at each subsequent expression. Your body will respond, as it does with the supply-and-demand let-down reflex. The amount of milk that can be expressed varies greatly with the individual. Some women have enough milk to donate to milk banks and others have just a few ounces. The amount of milk you are able to express, however, has nothing to do with your value as a mother. Some women become painfully depressed if they are able to express only a scanty amount of milk. Milk production has a great deal more to do with an individual's hormonal balance and the sucking nature of the infant (some infants have insatiable appetites, which ensure enormous milk production, and others are very casual in their eating habits) than it does with your maternal inclinations or your womanliness.

In addition to manual expression there are mechanical methods. You can use plastic suction pumps for the same purpose. These are composed of a rubber bulb and a plastic funnel.

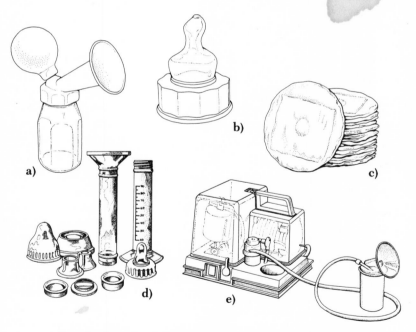

a) **Standard manual pump**   b) **NUK nipple**   c) **Breast pads**
d) **The Marshall pump**   e) **The electric pump**

The wide end of the funnel is placed over your areola. When you squeeze the bulb, a vacuum is created in the funnel, causing your milk to secrete. Personally, I find this method rather tiresome. The milk secretion is slow and the suction created is often so strong that it stings.

In my opinion, the best mechanical alternative is the Marshall hand pump. You can purchase one from a pharmaceutical or baby-supply store for about $20. These pumps are both efficient and highly portable (unlike the more cumbersome electric pumps), and consist of two high-impact cylinders that a working mother can take with her daily, ensuring an adequate supply of breast milk. The other alternative is the Egnell or Medella breast pump. These pumps are both electric and can be rented either from a pharmacy or from individuals for about $2 per day. Purchase of electric pumps is not generally recommended, since they are extremely expensive (about $600) and they are nonportable unless you have access to a car. If you feel you must purchase this kind of pump because you are unable to be with your child for long periods of time, you must purchase it directly from the manufacturer.

No matter how you choose to express your milk, always be sure to store it in a clean glass or plastic jar. If you plan to use it within four hours, you can keep it in the refrigerator. (*Note:* Milk will have to be heated to room temperature before a feeding.) If you wish to store it longer, you will have to freeze it, since it will spoil if kept for periods longer than four hours under normal refrigeration. Pour your milk into a clean plastic ice-cube tray and freeze it. When you are ready to use it, take a small saucepan filled with about an ounce of water (to dilute the milk) and heat the water on top of the stove. Place one or two "ice cubes" of your milk into the water. Heat until the cubes are thawed and then pour into a clean bottle. Many pediatricians recommend using the NUK Sanger nipples when bottle-feeding breastmilk, since their operation is more like the breast's than other manufactured nipples. If you are planning to bottle-feed your child during the night, simply leave a cube of frozen milk in the saucepan before you retire. This way the milk will be thawed by the time you are ready to use it.

One of the nicest things about bottle-feeding breast milk is that the father can take part and be one of the primary nurturers (see Chapter Six). Men don't often have the opportunity to become as close to their infants as mothers do, and although the husbands of mothers who are breast-feeding their babies are often proud and supportive of their wives' decision, there are many husbands who may feel jealous or even cheated because they don't share the closeness of association that breast-feeding brings. A young infant responds primarily to being fed. The new father may actually enjoy the chore of feeding his child, even if he has to perform it at three A.M. I feel it is desirable, if not absolutely necessary, that an infant form a close nurturing relationship with both parents.

You don't always have to express your milk if you want to get out of the house. A small breast-feeding infant is extremely portable. Family vacations are simple—no bottles or stale formula to worry about. You can go to a restaurant or even a movie and still breast-feed your child comfortably. If you are self-conscious, you can place a napkin or handkerchief over your breast. In many cases, a squealing infant can draw far more attention to you than breast-feeding will. If you are out shopping and your baby demands a feeding, simply go into the ladies' room. It is wise to learn of several accessible rest rooms if you plan to be out for several hours. The best rewards of outings with your infant are your own freedom. Staying at home and staring at four walls can create more stress than a couple of hours of brisk walking.

Though I discuss the working mother in more detail in Chapter Five, I feel that a brief discussion of the employee breast-feeding her child is due here. There is no reason for the mother to remain home. You can work and breast-feed your baby successfully. However, it is not a simple task. It requires planning, support, and physical and emotional stamina. My working situation during the postpartum period was very peculiar because I worked in an exercise studio which catered to both pregnant and postpartum mothers. I had the luxury of bringing my baby to work and nursing her there. There were also many other nursing mothers in my workplace, so I never felt uncomfortable. Unfortunately, this kind of working environment is extremely rare. If you happen to be a physician, a nurse, or a midwife, or happen to be employed in a day-care center, you are fortunate. Hospitals and care centers almost always provide on-site care for their employees' children. There are also some factories and large corporations that are beginning to establish on-site care in lieu of tax deductions for an improved attendance record of their female employees. The average woman, however, is unable to bring her infant to work with her unless she makes some special arrangement with her employer.

The next best alternative for an employee breast-feeding her baby is to find a licensed infant-care center close to your place of employment. You can breast-feed the baby in the morning, bring him to the care center, work for three to four hours, and then take a long lunch break during which you can visit the care center and again breast-feed your child. You can then return to work, finish your working day, and return to the care center in time for your baby's next feeding. This procedure can also work if you are employed relatively close to home. If these situations are not the case, you will have to express your milk manually or pump your breasts at regular intervals during your working day (about every three to four hours). Of course, this requires adequate refrigeration at your workplace. I recommend keeping your breast milk in a Thermos in the refrigerator and emptying it into an ice-cube tray when you return home. Use a manual or electric breast pump after dinner and before you go to sleep. In this manner, you can create an adequate supply of breast milk to leave with your baby-sitter on the following working day.

In Caribbean societies, where the mother almost always breast-feeds her child and works outside the home, the mother actually trains her baby to nurse through the night and sleep all day. In this manner, the breast-feeding infant sucks at his mother's breast only when she returns from work and sleeps during the day, while she is unavailable to suckle him. I have not, however, been able to find a single American woman who has practiced this. Personally, though I have never tried it, I feel it is rather drastic. The mother seems to receive little or no rest; she is working hard all day and nursing her child all night.

One important factor that the employee breast-feeding her baby must take into consideration is stress. Though stress and daily irritations will not "spoil your milk," as your grandmother may intimate, they will reduce its quantity. The stress of a demanding career can be overpowering even if you are not breast-feeding your baby. This, combined with the complications of new motherhood, can make your milk supply rather scanty. Do not allow this to discourage you, however. Continue to give breast milk as often as you can (one feeding a day is better than none at all) and supplement it with a nutritious formula, if necessary.

Another option, although it is not often practiced anymore in Western countries, is to use a wet nurse. Wet nurses, still used at the beginning of this century, are lactating mothers hired, usually by new mothers from the upper class, for the specific purpose of nursing their babies for them. The concept of having another woman nurse your baby is still followed in a few American rural communities, in which a kind of cooperative nursing circuit is developed among several women in a given neighborhood. If a mother needs to leave her nursing baby for any reason, she simply gives it to a neighboring lactating mother to feed. Perhaps the reason this nursing method is employed infrequently in the United States is that many American women, due to their social upbringing, have a culturally inbred aversion to sharing their babies' nursing with another woman. But the point is that, with sufficient planning, a mother nursing her child can maintain a relatively normal schedule, which can include a career and outside interests.

BODY IMAGE AND YOUR BREASTS

Because of the American cultural obsession with the breast, many women's feelings about their bodies change as a result of their decision to breast-feed their babies. As I have stated in Chapter One, a woman's perception of herself is often rooted in how she feels about her body. The breast, in our culture, has always had some expectations attached to it. In certain periods, it has been fashionable to be bosomy; in others, breasts have been literally bound, to appear nonexistent. The breast has largely been considered a sexual organ and not a nurturing one. The exposing of a naked breast to nurse a child in a public place is terrifying to some women. And, as far as some people are concerned, a woman who chooses to expose herself in this manner may as well be completely nude. New fathers may be horrified that their wives are revealing something previously reserved for them to anyone who may choose to look on. Remember, we have been brought up in a culture where breasts have little function except to intrigue the opposite sex. Though a previously small-breasted woman may take delight in her new shape, an amply endowed mother breast-feeding her child may suddenly see herself as overly seductive or indecent. The let-down reflex may also disturb some women; they may view breast milk as an excretion and associate it with other elimination processes.

These cultural attitudes may result in the average mother who is breast-feeding her child feeling repulsed by and ashamed of her nurturing function. Unfortunately, these perceptions of the breast and of breast-feeding have been slow to change. The slightly raised eyebrows of restaurant employees and of passersby in the park at the sight of a mother nursing her child may indeed be enough to influence the new mother into thinking that what she is doing is immodest and distasteful.

If you do feel this way (even the most confident of women may feel this way at some time), try to examine why carefully. If you find that it is mainly your environment that is making you uncomfortable—interfering relatives, disapproving glances, and so on, try to persevere. Avoid those situations that are unsupportive. For instance, if there is a restaurant that does not welcome your nursing your baby, don't go there; there will be many eating places that will accept breast-feeding.

If, however, you are truly uncomfortable about yourself, your breasts, and the whole concept of nursing, most doctors will recommend that you discontinue. To continue may mean that you will develop a very thwarted relationship with your infant. Remember, your whole concept of yourself should be integrated enough so that you are not overly concerned with your breasts and their function. Excessive concern can produce what I call the "milk machine" complex. Some new mothers begin to associate their entire personality with how their breasts are functioning.

During the past forty years, our culture has become so removed from natural breast functioning that the breast has come to represent something quite other than that for which it was intended. Your breasts are not merely the ingredients for playboy pictorials, they are a genuine part of your body—no more or less valuable than any other body part. If you can learn to view your breasts on an equal plane with the rest of yourself, you are well on your way to establishing the healthy body image so necessary to successful breast-feeding.

STAYING FIRM: BREAST AND PECTORAL EXERCISES

If there is a body part producing more anxiety in women than any other, it is surely the breast. This may be due to the fact that as far as the size and shape of our breasts are concerned, there is little we can do unless we resort to surgery. It is interesting to note that no matter what a woman's breasts may be like in reality, no woman ever sees her breasts as being exactly the correct size; they seem either too big or too small. There is, however, one characteristic that can be influenced—by proper exercise—and that is firmness. The pectoral muscles located underneath the breast tissue can be strengthened and toned, and they can help improve the appearance of your breasts. This is especially important for mothers nursing their babies, since the increased weight of the breasts will strain the pectoral muscles and cause premature sagging.

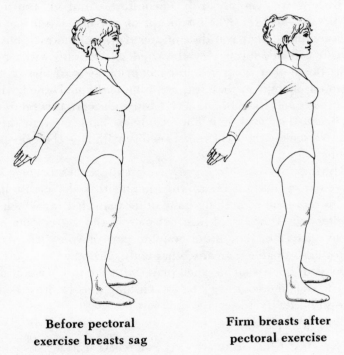

Before pectoral exercise breasts sag

Firm breasts after pectoral exercise

The following five exercises will keep your breasts firm and well toned. (*Note:* All of the exercises strengthen the pectoral muscles.)

The Press

This exercise can be performed in virtually any position (standing, sitting, lying down). Take a rubber ball and clasp it with both hands so that your fingers are laced over the top and your palms are parallel to each other. Lift your elbows so that they are in a parallel line with your shoulders. Press the ball together with the palms of your hands and hold for a slow count of three. Release. Repeat this exercise ten times.

Elbows

This exercise can be performed either sitting or standing. Stretch both of your arms directly in front of you, your hands parallel to your shoulders. Bend your elbows so that one of your hands lies directly on top of the other slightly under your chin. Now you are ready to begin. Sharply bring your elbows as far back as you can. Return to the beginning position. This exercise should be done rapidly—one count for each repetition. Do this exercise thirty times.

The Reach

Start on your hands and knees. Keeping your right arm straight, lift it laterally to shoulder level. Turn your head to the right and completely rotate your torso so that your arm is stretched as far behind you as possible. Slowly return to the beginning position. Repeat this sequence using your left arm. Complete this exercise eight times with each arm.

Push Away

Stand about two feet away from a wall, facing it, with your feet together. Place your hands on the wall at shoulder level. Slowly bend your elbows and bring your face as close to the wall as you can without moving your feet. Straighten your elbows and return to the beginning position. Repeat this exercise eight times.

The Big Circle

Stand erect with your legs about two feet apart and your arms at your sides. Raise both of your arms to shoulder level, then overhead, behind you, and then back to your sides. You should create momentum doing this so that you create a swinging motion. Repeat this exercise ten times.

Whether or not you decide to nurse your baby, you should remember that your baby's nutrition is of utmost importance. While mothers nursing their babies have reported a wonderful intimacy with them, due to the particular physical closeness of the nursing process, mothers not breast-feeding their babies can also achieve this kind of relationship, through a commitment to loving and cuddling their babies during feedings. Your choice of feeding methods is up to you. The previous information has been given to aid you in making this important decision.

Working Mother or Full-Time Mother: Options

Though much of what I have written in the previous chapters has a "how-to" flavor, this chapter is going to be slightly different. My reason for a more subjective, less practical approach here is that the nature of the material is broader. While there are precise guidelines to follow when discussing such tangible issues as nutrition, exercise, and anatomy, in researching styles of mothering, I found advice and information for two fundamentally different modes of mothering—that of traditional, or specifically child-oriented, mothering; and that of dual, or career/child-oriented, mothering. In either case, the attitudes toward the alternative, rather than specific instructions on being successful, appear to be the determining factor. My research shows that there is no single lifestyle that ensures becoming a "good" mother. What *is* significant in determining successful mothering is the way a particular woman feels about her chosen lifestyle, rather than the actual choice itself. Though I have included some practical information, such as how to evaluate a child-care center, most of the information here is centered on life-management skills that are not integral to your mothering role. In other words, specific advice, such as how to divide household chores, may make your day-to-day life simpler but will not necessarily make you a good or a bad mother.

The first point I want to emphasize is that I do not like the terms "working" and "nonworking." The woman who chooses to be a full-time homemaker and mother definitely works. However, the term "working mother" has come to mean a mother who earns a salary, whether she stays at home to do this or works outside the home. The term "nonworking" seems to render the traditional mother's lifestyle less valuable than the mother's who is said to be "working." Therefore, I have made a compromise. Though I will use the previously mentioned terms in certain contexts, in many instances I use other terminology to characterize these two alternative lifestyles. They are: "salaried" and "unsalaried"; "traditional" and "career"; and "wage-earning" and "non–wage-earning." I feel that these terms are more just, especially in regard to the mother who has chosen the traditional role.

Though much of this chapter deals specifically with the complications of the working mother, I did not choose to do this in order to diminish the role of the full-time mother. The reason is that most of us are the daughters of more traditional mothers. When we choose the role that parallels our mothers', we rear our children and keep our homes in very much the same manner that our mothers did. However, when we choose to be working mothers, we often have no role models, and as a result are often confused and insecure about the choice. In this chapter I will discuss each of these roles in the hope that you may identify yourself and thus be more able to prepare yourself for your new commitments.

"BEFORE I MET YOUR FATHER . . ." TRADITION, DISCRIMINATION, AND SEX STEREOTYPES

Most traditional mothers worked outside the home at one time. They went to college and even to graduate school. They became teachers, nurses, librarians, and secretaries. Some of them attained venerable awards in athletics and the arts. But this was all accomplished in that mythical period entitled "before I met your father. . . ." It is an interesting and enlightening comment on our society that many young girls equal and even surpass young boys in both scholastic and athletic abilities, yet once they reach puberty, they often automatically put these aspirations aside in preparation for building up the male ego. In a school in which I recently taught, I questioned the physical-education instructor on the progress of a certain gymnast. "Oh, she no longer comes to practice," he responded. "What happened?" I inquired in amazement. "What happens to all of the girls," he answered. "She fell in love."

In 1976, Helen Harris Solomons,[1] a noted psychologist, studied the coeducational physical-education programs in the Pennsylvania public schools. Though in the fifth-grade classes the results of specific tests designed to measure physical abilities demonstrated an equal number of boys and girls who were skilled, both the boys and the girls in these classes considered the boys to be superior. When a skilled girl achieved a higher score than a particular boy, she often attributed this higher score to pure luck rather than to her own superior ability. Boys, on the other hand, almost never attributed their achievements to luck rather to skill. This study seems to confirm that women are culturally induced from an extremely early age to believe that they are less gifted than men. Perhaps it has been women's long-standing acceptance of this myth, coupled with the belief that women do not have to prepare themselves for a career or become skilled because men will support them, that has led to the equally long-standing job discrimination against them, especially the wage-earning mothers of infants and young children.

Although the boards of education in nearly all U.S. states refused to hire married school teachers during the 1930s, most recently marriage itself has not been a cause for discrimination in the workplace. Pregnancy and subsequent childbirth are.

During the 1950s and the early 1960s, more than 60 percent of all wage-earning women were dismissed from their positions when pregnancy was discovered. Thanks to an amendment to Title VII of the Civil Rights Act of 1964, which outlawed discrimination on account of pregnancy, such practices are now illegal in most states in this country. Today, you will find a large number of healthy pregnant women working in all occupations.

However, job situations offer no such guarantees for the postpartum mother. There are no laws in this country specifically protecting from job discrimination the mother who chooses to work outside the home. The wage-earning mother in today's society is subject to less overt, far subtler forms of prejudice than the early feminists were. The first misconception is the notion that most of the female population stays home with the children while the husbands work. According to 1976 statistics, 54 percent of all American mothers with preschool children earned a salary, and that percentage continues to increase. The second and perhaps most damaging myth is that women do not need to work. The fact is that most American mothers earning wages need their money to support their families. Continuing inflation makes the luxury of one breadwinner per family a fact of the past. Many families formerly able to get by on one salary now need the purchasing power of two salaries to beat the rising cost of inflation. The most current statistics[2] indicate that the average cost of raising a child to maturity when only one parent works is about $98,000 for the first child and $48,000 for each subsequent child. Currently, only 34 percent of all American households are supported by the husbands alone. There is also an increasing number of single women having babies. Eleven percent of all firstborn American children are not the result of a legal marriage. The women who give birth to these children will have to head and support their own households. While there has always been a small percentage of women giving birth to children out of wedlock, as well as widows and poor women who are forced to work to support their children, the more recent influx of middle-class working mothers into the labor force has drastically changed the traditional view of marriage and family over the past twenty years.

Even though women have a great need for economic security, they continue to be discriminated against. This is doubly so for the mothers of small children. A single mother of a preschool child—due to the expense of private day care, the lack of public day care, and sex discrimination—is six times more likely to be earning below the United States poverty level than a person in any other segment of American society. Economic stability has a tremendous effect on the health and welfare of our children. High unemployment rates and the resulting poverty are often the causes of alcoholism, drug addiction, and child abuse. Economic stress may hinder effective parenting.

Financial stress is not only an economic issue but also a social and psychological issue. The fact is that although our society may see the traditional mothering role as a necessity, unless our economic system changes, most women will need to work even while their children are infants. Economists predict that, with the annual inflation rate of 10 percent at this writing, a predominating pattern of two-income families will emerge.

Because of this economic trend, women need to take a serious look at the way they view themselves as providers and at the way they see themselves combining this role with mothering.

Many women today do not wish to identify with the traditional mothering role:

> *My mother lived in a vacuum. She lived her life through us and we all suffered for it. I always loved my mother yet I can't say I respected her contributions to society.*

There are several studies that indicate that women who identify strongly with their fathers, rather than with their mothers, tend to have higher self-esteem than their mother-identifying counterparts. Marjorie Lozoff, of the Wright Institute at Berkeley, conducted an interesting experiment.[3] She found that if fathers, in particular, demonstrated a strong interest in the work abilities of their daughters—as opposed to the traits traditionally viewed as feminine, such as being pretty or being quiet—this kind of praise would result in noteworthy initiative and self-appreciation when these women reached maturity. Why are fathers so representative of self-esteem to young women? Because men's lives are so entwined with work and the outside world. In the American work ethic, earning wages is an accomplishment worthy of honor. Working and not getting paid for it is deemed as having less value than the same work that earns a salary. Because of this attitude, many more mothers now enter the workplace not only for financial reasons but for an improved self-image and sense of accomplishment.

Although childless women can also suffer discrimination in the workplace as a result of long-held cultural prejudices against working women in general, the mother of young children receives special scrutiny. Society condones the single, childless woman in the workplace to some degree because she doesn't have anyone else to support her. But the new mother who is working professionally is often seen either as neglecting her baby or as not having married well enough to be provided for. The longevity of this view of women's place in the workplace may be found in the history of the feminist movement in this country. Suffragettes at the turn of the century were more interested in obtaining the right to vote for women than in finding them an appropriate place in the work force, probably because many were sufficiently wealthy, or were unmarried scholars and writers, who at that time did not consider sex discrimination in labor the pressing issue. Later, in the 1960s, the new feminists, many of whose children had grown and left home, had the time to concentrate on developing their careers and wanted the opportunity to do so. However, in the 1980s, we, the daughters who were reared during the period of the 1960s feminist philosophy, are experiencing a new conflict— that of developing a career and raising a family at the same time, rather then deferring one for a time to concentrate on the other. Being first a full-time mother and then a breadwinner, after the children are grown, is a simpler alternative and is considered a more respectable one than trying to integrate these two life components simultaneously.

However, in one University of Michigan study,[4] evidence was presented to indicate that "definite work plans" were significant in diminishing the depression that often accompanies childbirth. Thus, the integration of career and mothering is not only desirable, but a criterion for mental health. It may interest social scientists that the "sacred" isolation of the mother–infant dyad is a fairly recent phenomenon in history. This concept did not arise until the eighteenth century and the Industrial Revolution. Historically, women and their young children were not separated from the workings of society. Women in rural communities were sweating in the fields and shopkeepers' wives were weighing flour while their infants were still nursing. The separation began as industry grew and new mothers, concerned over the health of their babies in factory environments, began to take piecework home with them. However, they couldn't complete their work as quickly by hand as they could by machine and so were soon laid off. As a result, industry stopped hiring new mothers and began to terminate employment of women who became pregnant. This vicious practice trailed into the twentieth century.

In a number of other cultures, women and their children are not left isolated from the workplace as we are in the United States. In many primitive cultures, male parental investment is high if women's work is considered as important as the men's. For example, if the division of labor in a given culture dictates that the women grow the crops or vegetables, the men of the tribe will often be seen gathered in a closely knit group fondling and singing to their children while their wives work in the fields. When the men go hunting, the women assume the nurturing role. It is interesting that in tribes that practice this equal division of labor and parenting, there is little evidence of sex stereotypes. Male children are not trained in warlike behavior, because war, interestingly enough, is practically nonexistent in these cultures, and the female children are not taught to be subservient to the men.

Anthropologists have termed societies where there is an absence of sex stereotypes as "androgynous." The term "androgynous" means having both male and female characteristics; as applied to societies, however, it denotes a culture in which there is a high degree of sexual equality. The fundamental aspect of androgynous societies is deep mutual respect between sexual partners. And postpartum recovery in these cultures—though there may not be a specific term for it in a given language—is recognized through actions as a time in which the mother is under extraordinary pressure. During his wife's postpartum recovery, a husband in an androgynous society will often sleep with his older children, exclusively caring for them during the day so that his wife may care for and nurse the new baby. One such androgynous society is that of the bushmen of northern Botswana. Their essentially agrarian economy provides a natural environment for sharing parenting. The parents literally share the work in this society, each parent devoting half of the week to farming and/or hunting and the other half to the care and nurturing of their children. This society also provides a time slot for leisure so that both parents can be with their children at the same time. It is also interesting that in societies such as this one there is no divorce, no extramarital sexual partnering. A person chooses a sex partner for life. It seems that mutual respect for each other's role in society may create monogamy. There is also an astounding correlation between a society's understanding and acceptance of postpartum recovery as a special period and that society's view of women's work contribution to that particular society. In other words, if a woman is seen only as a nurturer of children, especially of male children, and not identified also as a vegetable grower, a weaver, or a breadmaker, her biological functions—which include postpartum recovery—are often made to seem trivial.

Androgynous social structure exists also in several modernized countries, such as Sweden, mainland China, the Soviet Union, and Israel. These countries, due largely to the socialistic nature of their government, which requires all people to work, have enacted legislation to provide for total sexual equality and government-subsidized day care. I will discuss later in this chapter the methods by which the United States could attain an androgynous social structure.

In the United States where sex stereotypes are prevalent, the demeaning of women's work has moved the social roles of men and women further apart emotionally as well as geographically. The less similar the roles of men and women are in a given society, the less social identification they will share with one another. During American pioneering times, although women did not legally have the right to vote or to own property in the wilderness, this particular civil-rights issue did not seem to matter. A man needed his wife to run his farm, to breed chickens, and to sell the eggs in the marketplace. If she was laid up with child or had a bad case of "milk fever," it was a crucial problem. Her needs were attended to so that she could get back out into the fields and help the family survive economically. More recently in our culture, however, women and children have not been viewed as a financial necessity but rather as a financial burden on the man who might have to support them. The more a woman is seen as a burden, the less right she is given to complain about her biological discomforts.

However slowly, in American society the pendulum in now beginning to swing away from this biased view of the mother. Though many women need to value themselves in the traditional role of primary nurturer, the right—not to mention the economic and psychological need—of the mothers of infants and small children to work outside the home has become a fundamental issue. Wage earning is an integral part of the way a woman values herself. In 1976, The University of Michigan[5] conducted a study that reviewed the attitudes of American teenagers. Only 11 percent of the girls interviewed saw themselves in the future primarily as housewives; 72 percent of the girls and 76 percent of the boys saw their future careers as being "central" to their lives. Even if given a circumstance in which they would not have to work, such as marrying a rich man or inheriting a fortune, 84 percent of the girls said that they would want to work anyway. The same girls viewed marriage and family with equal intensity. Only 6 percent rejected the idea of marriage; 61 percent wanted to become mothers within their first two years of marriage. These young girls saw balancing a career and mothering not only as a possibility but as a necessity for developing themselves as complete persons.

Gail Sheehy, in her famous book *Passages*,[6] about the stages of adult development, coined a word for women who choose to merge marriage, career, and children simultaneously, rather than postponing a career until their families are raised or doing the reverse by postponing a family until their careers are established. She calls these women, not surprisingly, "integrators." Sheehy discovered in her research that, although "integrating" is emotionally very difficult for women in their early twenties, the prospect of "integrating" at ages twenty-eight to thirty becomes highly possible. True integrators do not leave the work force to raise their children. They may take a short leave but, essentially, they "hang in" there. Sheehy considers herself and many other successful women "integrators." My feeling, as an integrator, is that a career and the self-esteem it creates enhances mothering and that the intimacy and communication that mothering provides enhances your work.

American society's view of the career mother with small children is rapidly improving. In 1977, the *New York Times*[7] reported that 75 percent of all young men between the ages of eighteen and twenty-nine wanted their wives to work outside the home even when they had children. This statistic nearly matched the response of the young women in the same age group.

It is true that women are having fewer children today and at a decidedly later age. Statistically, a professional woman spends at least seven years in the workplace before she chooses to marry and bear children. But new mothers are not leaving their positions for as long as they once did (which was often permanently). Almost 40 percent of all new mothers return to their jobs before their baby is a year old, and that number is growing. This circumstance requires a new understanding on the part of both employers and employees about the psychological and social implications of postpartum recovery. This, in turn, will demand the reversal of some of our most inbred sex stereotypes and will require not only legislation for equal opportunity but also a real psychological commitment from both men and women to establish a standard for shared parental and career responsibilities.

". . . And What Do You Do?" The Unsalaried Career

All of a sudden you are "just a mother." It is kind of like being called an outcast. I worked for a long time in the business world and I enjoy being home with my baby now. I don't feel that it will be a permanent decision but, for the time being, I want to be recognized for having made the right choice for myself.

Liberal feminists today believe that homemaking is fine as long as it is "your choice" and not something arrived at through male pressure. However, women making this choice may feel belittled by some feminists because they may feel they are being merely patronized and not truly accepted.

I believe that while staying home with small children is a logical direction for many mothers to take, it must be done with the realization that you are not always going to be a full-time mother. Your children will grow up and leave home, most of them before you are fifty years old, and therefore you will have a good twenty to thirty years of living to do without them. Taking a new career direction at fifty or even at forty can be difficult. In my opinion, it is much more logical to cultivate other life interests while you are mothering so that you do not become the victim of the common "empty nest" syndrome.

A woman who chooses mothering and homemaking as full-time commitment will normally perform a variety of work tasks during her day. Changing diapers, heating cereal, and folding laundry is certainly work by any standard. Our society, however, views this work as less valuable than filling cavities, ordering a shipment of pantyhose, or designing a breakfast cereal box. If a woman chooses to use a skill traditionally viewed as feminine—say, baking cheesecake—and selling the product to restaurants for profit, then her working status is higher because she is being paid for what she is doing. Making a cheesecake at home for the family is simply not seen as a prestigious task. Women are being given double messages here. Stay home with your children because that is what you are expected to do, but don't expect to be admired for doing so.

Several recent sociological[8] studies have indicated that school-age girls regard their mothers as making the same contribution to the family as their fathers only if their mothers had outside jobs. The most intriguing factor about the children involved in this study is that both the boys and the girls of career mothers wanted their fathers, not their mothers, home more often. They also wanted their fathers to help their career mothers with the household chores more often so that their mothers would not be so tired. There was no such concern expressed from the children of the traditional mothers. It was assumed by these children that it was the mother's duty to carry the entire household load. Though unintentionally, we may be passing the low-status notion of the traditional mother on to our children.

"So what do I do?" you ask. "Get a job just so that I'm ensured respect?" Not necessarily. First, you need to have a talk with your husband, preferably before or while you are still pregnant. Try to establish what your expectations are going to be for yourself and from each other. Let it be known that you do not want to become a maidservant. Make your expectations as clear as possible. You certainly do not want to end up like one of those striking housewives we have heard of lately. These women seemCnto have been tramped on by their husbands and children, while their own interests have been completely ignored. Finally, they are revolting and thereby beginning to assemble some respect for themselves. In a marriage where you and your husband understand and respect each other, your children grow up in a positive atmosphere. You also need to talk to some full-time mothers, to learn what their experiences have been and how you might incorporate their suggestions into your own family life.

Total economic dependence on men had a tremendous psychological impact on women throughout history. Women marrying in the late 1940s and early 1950s, and mothering the baby boom, were raised to believe that their husbands would and should take care of them. Working was the refuge of the unfortunate woman who had married poorly, who was unmarried, or who was sadly widowed. During the early 1960s, feminists sprang up protesting the traditional female role. There were goals for higher education and job opportunities, and for legislation about birth control; there were symbolic displays of liberation such as bra burnings. The juxtaposition of the traditional and the radical views of women in society may have been confusing but certainly allowed women a wider range of choices than had been previously available.

People began to notice that some of the gilded images of family life and motherhood were not necessarily true ones. Husbands and wives divorced. Husbands became unemployed. Women, who traditionally live far longer than men, became widowed with no marketable skills and sometimes with children to support. The idea that perhaps women had better educate themselves "just in case" became more prevalent. We often see older women at the cashier counter or waiting endlessly on tables in a diner. These women may be the ones who were sold the "American dream." True, work of any kind has dignity, but many of these older women have to resort to low-paying jobs because they have no skills with which to support themselves after their husbands are gone. So, because of these pressing realities, many women began to educate themselves not just as insurance against crises but as a means of establishing themselves as people.

There are many reasons for women to choose to be full-time mothers. There are many women who perform nurturing skills extremely well and may be better off, if they can afford it, to stay home with their young children rather than to take an outside job. Other women, after having spent a number of years in the work force, simply want a change:

> I've been working on Wall Street for almost eight years. My husband has finally finished his training and set up in his own office. We planned this baby and I want to take some time off. I don't have any definite plans about returning to work because I want to have a second child relatively soon. I'm not even sure if I want to return to Wall Street, and switching careers right now just doesn't seem practical to me.

Situations like this are not uncommon. Many women want the experience of "just being a mother":

> Jeff and I are having only one child. We decided that even before we got married. This is the only opportunity I'll have to be a mother and I want to take advantage of it.

The important factor to remember in establishing yourself in the traditional role is not to lose your identity. This statement may sound like popular psychology but it is valid. You are not going to be a new mother forever, and to live your own life through your child's may cause great unhappiness for both of you. Develop yourself; your education does not end when you become a mother. Go to the library; take those sculpture classes you always wanted to. Use this "time off" as a kind of sabbatical. Your life deserves to grow and thrive so that you do not become an unfulfilled and bored housewife when you arrive at mid-life. As a woman, you may have to face the unhappy yet ultimate truth that it is very likely that you will be completely alone someday. Since men's life expectancy is shorter than women's, it's doubly important to learn self-sufficiency—whether intellectual or financial—now, not later, when it may be too late.

"Of Course, I'm Going Back to Work"

Look into the eyes of many healthy, career-oriented pregnant women, and they will tell you that the alternative of staying home after their babies are born has simply never crossed their minds. They have worked hard to get to where they are, and although they can't wait to take on their mothering duties, they are resuming their outside career as soon as possible. The casualness with which they say this indicates to me that most pregnant women don't envision the true commitment to an infant that is necessary. You can't just plop an infant on top of your desk, go on with your work, and smile at him at regular intervals. A child is not like a pet. And, although taking your baby to work with you is often cited as being the ideal solution for the career mother, you may not want to plan an advertising campaign with a toddler hugging your leg. Being a mother is a job that requires the same level of commitment that any other profession does.

The young mothers of the 1980s are perhaps the first generation of middle-class American women who have seriously considered combining motherhood with their chosen professions. Immigrant women, women living in agricultural communities, and poor women (before there was welfare) have always worked. They had no choice. They worked or they starved. Even today, almost 70 percent of all working mothers in the United States are either the sole support for their children or have husbands who do not earn an income adequate to support the family's lifestyle. However, women do not assume their role as providers in the same manner that men do. We rarely read stories, though they are becoming more frequent, about how men manage to keep both a family and a career intact. Traditionally men have not considered this notion. However responsible a man may see himself in regard to his family, to him the family is still his wife's priority. He may be financially responsible, but he does not see himself emotionally responsible for his family as often as his wife may. Hence, the average mother, no matter how crucial her paycheck may be to her family's financial stability, may still leave the house every morning feeling guilty. Adding to the emotional conflict is the fact that many employers are not very helpful in helping a woman integrate mothering with her career. Often, she may be expected to be married to her profession and leave the mothering side of herself at the threshold of the office door. Due to her cultural upbringing, however, this severing of the mothering from the professional side of herself is never entirely possible. Her superior, especially if he is a man, simply may not be able to empathize with her conflict. She may end up feeling indebted to her family and to her job and never being able to satisfy either one or, for that matter, herself.

There are several factors to consider if you choose to return to work. The first is timing—when to do it? Can you afford to remain home for six months, a year, longer? Do you want to stay home for that long? I am convinced that there is no single correct time to return to outside work. I have known women who returned to their professions three days after delivery and others who waited five years. Some women, confident during pregnancy, tell their employers that they will return in three to six months and then find, for a variety of reasons, that they simply are unable to do so. Other women, confident in their job security during their pregnancy, try to return to their jobs a year later only to find that their positions have been taken or that the nature of their jobs has changed. Many of these women have had to go to court for the sake of principle. This is sad because all that most of them want is their jobs— they don't want a fight. It is also a sad comment on our society, which says that, if you want to become a mother, you may have to lose your place on the career-advancement ladder.

But more important than timing is the nature of your work situation. Is your work situation compatible with your decision to become a parent? There are several things to consider when evaluating a workplace. Does your work environment provide child care? Though most work situations do not provide this service, if your particular company does, it is a definite plus for any working mother. Do you have flexible hours? This is probably the most significant factor in evaluating a work environment. Unfortunately, the typical structure of the American workday leaves a great deal to be desired. In most corporate and professional environments, hours are so rigidly structured that they can severely limit our time as mothers. We come home from work so exhausted that we cannot possibly take adequate time to be nurturers. The very obvious solution to this dilemma may be either to work fewer hours or to take extra work home with you. Discuss these alternatives with your employer. Let him or her know that as a new mother you will have new responsibilities and that you will want every opportunity to perform both jobs reasonably well. Another solution may be to work close to home so that you can have that two-hour commuting time to spend with your family.

Another question to consider is what your company's policy is on families. This may sound like a strange question but it is extremely important. Basically, can your superior accept the fact that you are a family member with responsibilities not related to work and not "just a worker"?

My boss became an entirely different person when I became a mother. He suggested that I behave like the men in our company, who behaved as if they had no loyalties outside of their jobs. I found his attitude painfully unfair.

For instance, you wake up one morning and your daughter has a fever. You cannot find a sitter on the spur of the moment and you cannot take her to the day-care center in that condition. Do you call your boss and tell him or her the truth, or do you make an excuse? If you feel that you would have to make an excuse or if you feel that if you told the truth you would elicit an unsympathetic response, it may be a good idea to talk seriously with your employer before this common situation arises. In the future, there may be nonemergency events in which you would like to participate. Your daughter may have a basketball game or a daytime music recital that you may want to attend. Child-oriented institutions, which include schools, hospitals, and social-welfare agencies, tend to be particularly empathetic toward family situations. Large corporations, which women have only recently infiltrated, are more difficult. Also, if there are no other mothers in your work environment, you may be setting a precedent. No one will be sure just how to react to you. You may be being tested by your male colleagues to see if you are going to "cut it" once you become a mother.

It is also wise to consider your situation economically. Does your job pay well enough? Would it be in your future interest to educate or train yourself in another profession, which has a superior earning capacity? In this manner, you could work fewer hours, secure yourself financially, and still have ample time to be a parent.

How much time is necessary? No one knows for sure, but in a 1977 study,[9] more than one third of the children of working mothers interviewed felt that they wanted their mothers to spend more time with them. Perhaps it is the quality of the time that is significant in determining effective parenting and not just the number of hours spent with a child.

If you cannot find a job that is compatible with your responsibilities as a parent, you may find that creating your own job is the answer. One woman I know was a successful fashion consultant for a major department store. She had been working in this profession for years and was committed to returning to her position three months after delivery of her baby. The three months' maternity leave turned into six months. She was afraid to return to her job because it required so much traveling that she would not have enough time for her daughter. She made the difficult decision to leave her job, one she enjoyed tremendously, and established her own fashion consulting business. She still has to travel occasionally for business reasons but now at least she feels it is her choice and not an employer's. My own decision to write professionally partially stemmed from not finding other suitable avenues through which to complete myself both as a mother and as a career woman.

That's having your own business, you say; doesn't that often require more time than working for someone else? Well, yes and no. It depends on what you elect to do and how you plan to do it. Taking on a partner is often helpful. In that manner, you can cover for each other. If you can operate from your home, it may be even better. By working at home, you can save the commuter time, too.

Perhaps the most essential ingredient to the management and planning of your time is the involvement of your husband. Although there are still some traditional husbands, who believe a "woman's place is in the home," many men now enjoy their wives' having the financial independence. It makes their own career ambitions less tense, more human:

I really admire my husband. He took initiative in his work environment. Taking time off after the baby was born and staying home two afternoons a weeks while I teach class was something unheard of in his office, and he was subject to a great deal of ridicule at first. But now other men, seeing the satisfaction Dick enjoys with his new baby, are asking for the same consideration. Perhaps if other men start insisting, workplaces would take on a different attitude.

Married couples need to understand that being a career-oriented husband or wife and being career-oriented parents are two different things. When a husband and wife have only each other to consider, life can be comparatively simple. When a third person arrives, he or she can temporarily tilt the balance of that relationship. Many husbands, like their wives, are unprepared for the responsibilities to an infant. Some husbands, unintentionally, will award the child-care arranging and the career manipulating solely to their wives under the presumption that nothing should interfere with a man's professional life.

This view is slowly changing. Men, previously locked into the rigidity of their jobs, long for the intimacy that family life offers. They want to spend more time with their wives and children. Their relatively new presence in the delivery room is evidence of this longing. In most experimental situations, men have proved again and again that they are just as loving a parent as any woman can be. More and more men are getting involved in the childrearing process. They are working four days a week or taking afternoons off or taking work home with them to finish after their children fall asleep. I see them in the park early in the morning with a stroller or seated, briefcase in hand, during an early afternoon gymnastics class. They are still few but at least they exist.

If you are planning to work outside the home, it is important to sit down with your husband and divide responsibilities. I feel that it is best to divide the work depending upon what one enjoys doing or what an individual is more capable of doing. The working hours for one of you may be more conducive to taking the baby to the day-care center, and those of the other more conducive to picking him or her up at the end of the workday. One person's job may offer such a flexibility of working hours that it may be more logical for him or her to do all of the chauffeuring. It doesn't really matter how you arrange your schedule so long as both of you feel you are obtaining adequate satisfaction from your professional and family lives and neither one of you feels that he or she is missing out on something vital.

Another issue to consider with your husband and with your friends is whether or not you like your job. This is of central concern especially during postpartum recovery, when your self-esteem is so crucial. If you continue to work in a non-supportive environment or in a profession that is not compatible with your abilities, your opinion of yourself is generally lowered. There are also instances in which the new mother may return to work and find that the profession that was compatible with her previous lifestyle is not compatible with her new role. Men will also often require career changes, but they don't consider this option after having a child as often as women do. If you begin to be or have been dissatisfied with your job, speak with your husband and see if the two of you can cooperate so that you can make the desired career change. This may mean taking time off from the work force and going back to school, but as a long-range goal, it may be worth it.

Do you feel guilty about working outside the home? Most mothers do. This is largely a result of concepts of American culture, which traditionally has considered the "working woman" unreliable due to her potential responsibilities as wife and mother. However, being the mother of an infant requires a set of skills that not all women have or enjoy performing. Not all women enjoy lullabies and peek-a-boo games. If you can hire someone who enjoys singing animal songs and playing finger games while you are out performing a skill in which you are proficient, you may actually be doing your child a service. Your skills may be more valuable at a later point in your child's development, such as being able to discuss economic modes for your child's civics class. Staying at home and being bored and resentful during the seemingly endless afternoons of cartoon reruns just to avoid feeling guilty is not going to promote the kind of loving relationship that both mothers and children need.

The children of working mothers, although they may want their mothers to be with them more often, do learn unconsciously to identify with their mother's work role. The daughters of immigrant women, for example, whose mothers were often forced into work roles for economic reasons, were found to be extraordinarily influenced by their mothers. Though the jobs held by these immigrant women were never held in high esteem, the women were often admired for their ability to earn a living. A recent study[10] has indicated a correlation between having an immigrant mother and being a successful careerwoman. If a child grows up recognizing his or her mother's work life, the child learns to respect her in a new way. She comes to reflect the outside world and its expectations. This situation is especially valuable to female children, who need to broaden their aspirations and perfect their abilities in this ever more competitive world.

The last but certainly not the least important issue to consider is your own ambition. Exactly what do you expect from your career and your family? American society has been very severe with its working mothers. In some instances women have had to barter advancement and salary increases to obtain greater flexibility in their work hours. Working mothers have often been kept in lower-paying, less desirable positions in the belief that, because their loyalties are divided, they will not be as conscientious in their work as their male counterparts. Many mothers with professions conscious of this attitude, try to over-compensate by becoming insensitive workaholics, as if the "work only" attitude of men was something to aspire to. You may also have to accept the reality, as your husband will have to if he is fully to share parenting with you, that you may not be able to compete with the man or the woman who, because of no attachments, is able to be completely work-oriented sixteen hours per day.

The attitude that work should be completely severed from family is extremely prejudiced and also unfounded. Studies indicate that work environments that provide for family concerns, by giving maternity and paternity leaves and by having on-site day-care centers, actually have less absenteeism, better morale, and a higher rate of production than those companies that insist that you behave like a schizophrenic—being totally a parent one moment and totally a worker the next. If you are truly a professional and truly value yourself as a person, you must sometimes insist that your priorities be respected. This may mean "rocking the boat" temporarily, but you can change a situation if you put your mind to it. As one woman has stated,

> *I was terrified of confronting my boss. He was in at seven-thirty* A.M. *every morning and sometimes didn't leave until after six* P.M. *I really felt that with my job and family obligations I had to leave the office regularly at four* P.M. *I was willing to take my work home with me and finish it after my baby fell asleep. When I met with him, I discussed my position, and to my amazement he just looked at me and said, "You know, you're right. I don't spend enough time with my family, either."*

In some instances, women will simply harbor their resentments, and supervisors will just assume that nothing is wrong. Discussion with your husband, your boss, and other mothers with careers is essential in developing a suitable career/parent balance.

The key words in combining career and motherhood seem to be flexibility and planning. American society, unfortunately, was not entirely prepared for the entrance of the mother who is also a career woman into the work force. Paid work in this country has been structured for the traditional lifestyle of men who leave parenting and household responsibilities to the unsalaried women at home. This has enabled men to develop a concentrated effort in their workplace devoid of any family concerns. This situation has come to be respected and sought after by employers. When a professional woman who is a mother enters the work force, her conflicts are magnified by her sex and her priorities. These circumstances can and must be altered not only for career women who are mothers but also for the husbands who may want to share parenting on an equal footing with their wives. The solution to this parenting/work conflict lies in businesses and individuals foreseeing new methods of implementing work skills in an environment more conducive to family interests. New parents often have to improvise. Their own parents didn't have similar conflicts so they have no mentors to follow. There are also many culturally sexist concepts deep in the heart of the most liberal of us—for example, the wife should do the laundry and the husband should pay the bills. Improvising of course involves the flexibility and planning to which I have previously referred. This is surely not an impossible task. The pressure of concerned parents has created solutions in other countries. Since 1976, Sweden has had a national policy about sick leave that includes the illness of children. Both parents are allowed time in which to stay home for a child's illness as well as for their own. Since 1970, Sweden has had a system of paid maternity and paternity leaves; the mother and father are allowed seven months' combined leave after the birth of a child, with 95 percent of their pay. In contrast, although there is maternity leave granted in most American employment, only 31 percent of American businesses offer paternity leave. As Letty Cottin Pogrebin stated before a Senate subcommittee on discrimination on account of pregnancy, "If men could get pregnant, maternity benefits would be as sacrosanct as the GI bill." Flexible work hours, which in European countries are provided for five million workers, affect only about 300,000 workers in the United States. Publicly subsidized day care is also a possible solution to the parent/career balancing problem. In almost all industrialized nations, such care is readily available. But that is not the case in this country. We are the only industrialized nation in the world that does not have a parenting or children's allowance built into our social security system. This allowance, which is available in many countries, is a federal subsidy given to the parents of young children. This subsidy is not viewed in the same manner as welfare or a "handout" but rather as a kind of insurance for families who may need it. The fear is that the implementation of such a subsidy will create overpopulation by encouraging women to have more children. It is interesting that in both France and the Soviet Union, where such a subsidy is offered, there has been no significant increase in family size as a result.

This kind of legislation, which has been enacted in other countries, should be initiated here in the United States. It will take initiative on the part of family members to make it a reality. As more parents demand recognition for their role as parents, society may move closer to more family-oriented work situations for all employed people.

THE CHILD-CARE GAME

One of the most intriguing factors I discovered in my research is that a very high percentage of American women classified as occupational successes were either foreign born or had at least one immigrant parent. Of course, there were other statistical factors included in the criteria for outstanding women achievers, such as being affluent or having had adequate role models, but why was being foreign born or having an immigrant parent so significant in predicting success?

Upon further investigation, I discovered that middle- and upper-class women in many foreign countries are not expected to take care of their children full time. They hire people to do this for them or enter their children in a child-care program, which is usually government funded. Even poorer immigrant women do not view full-time mothering as mandatory. When they come to this country, they usually have to work at substandard jobs to survive. Their children most naturally are placed in the care of another person. These women often encourage their daughters to get a good education so that later they will have good opportunities in the career market. Though this different attitude toward mothering is not prevalent in all foreign countries, most foreign-born women do not feel guilty about having their children cared for by someone else. The absence of the guilt factor makes it significantly easier for foreign-born women to enter traditionally male professions. There is an infinitely higher percentage of women architects, scientists, and engineers in foreign countries than in the United States.

From a certain point of view, even the poorer, less educated women in other industrialized nations have greater work opportunities than do American women. We are one of the few industrialized nations in the world with no form of nationwide day care. A low-income family in this country may face dire poverty when a child is born; the family may lose half of its income if the wife is unable to work. And let's face it, welfare is never adequate and often psychologically demeaning. At least, if a poor woman in a foreign country can find a job, she does not have to worry about her baby. The child will be placed in a government-licensed child-care center that provides nutritional food and stimulating, loving care. The status of foreign child-care workers is high. Their training is thorough, rigorous, and professional. Compare this with the typical child-care worker in the United States, who is often grossly underpaid and under-educated. This country has no equivalent to the child-care systems representative of most other industrialized nations. Although there are some free day-care centers in this country, they are often inadequate and even inhuman. The National Council of Jewish Women has conducted a nationwide survey of public day-care centers and has reported:

> Mothers leave their children in tears every morning at the center door, weeping because they know their children are being mistreated, but there is no place else to put them. Centers are presided over by the old, the blind, the mentally retarded, the simply dull; centers promise to toilet train toddlers and use suppositories to do so.[11]

Situations like this are appalling, and although this study was conducted in 1975, they still continue to exist. The irony of this situation is that our country boasts so heartily of the health and well-being of its children and yet continues to neglect their most basic needs. For every seven children in this country who need day care, only one will receive it; and only 25 percent of those mothers whose children are able to have day care are satisfied with their day-care situation.[12] The fact is that nation-wide day care is desperately needed in this country if we want to offer equal opportunity to all new mothers, regardless of status or income. My feeling is that the initiation of such programs is being deterred because of the long-held social prejudices against women in the workplace, especially the mothers of infants and small children. During World War II, our country rose to support women who worked outside the home because they were needed to hold the country together economically while the men were abroad. Women with infants and young children were no exception. A phenomenal nationwide day-care system was instituted, accompanied by official propaganda urging women to go to work for their country. The centers were clean and staffed with warm, educated teachers and students. There were plenty of good toys available and substantial food. What happened to these wonderful centers? They disappeared when the men came home, took over their previously held jobs, and pushed their women back into the home again.

It is also interesting to look at the media during the World War II period. During the war, women's magazines were filled with articles on how to make quick, nutritious meals for your children so that you wouldn't have to spend so much time cooking and would be more available to hold down a job. There were also articles on how well-provided your children would be in day-care centers. After the war was over, the same magazines featured recipes that took six hours to prepare and articles that reported on the damaging psychological effect of a mother's career on her children. It seems that, in American society, a woman's "place" is traditionally determined by where men choose to place her.

After my discussion of the negative realities of American child-care systems, it may be comforting for you to know that I am also prepared to report on some of the more adequate alternatives. It is unfortunate that many of these alternatives still depend upon your income. However, the realization of this problem may urge women as a group to demand further legislation on this issue and perhaps eradicate the ill-doings of the past.

The most common child-care arrangement in this country is to hire a person to come into your home expressly for this purpose. This method is also perhaps the most expensive (upwards of $150 per week), but it does offer certain conveniences. The child-care worker who comes to your home usually also performs the role of housekeeper and even of secretary in some cases. She or he can often alleviate many household pressures, in addition to caring for your child. When a family income is unable to support this particular kind of care, the most usual substitute has been one of the grandmothers or another close relative whom the family may not feel obligated to pay a salary. The present difficulty with the latter method is that very often the grandmother is working full time herself and is no longer available for free baby-sitting.

One drawback to the arrangement of hiring someone, in my opinion and in the opinion of many child professionals, is that unless the person you hire is especially gifted and educated, your child may not be receiving adequate stimulation at home. This may not matter initially, as a small infant needs more to be cuddled than given an intellectual discussion, but as your child reaches the age of eight to nine months, he or she begins to need the company of more people—other children, in particular, in order to be able to cope effectively with separation anxiety, which I will discuss fully in Chapter Six.

Another method of child-care practiced in this country is the informal family-care home. This form of care is largely unlicensed because in the United States, if people choose to care for fewer than seven children other than their own in their home on a regular basis, they are not required to be licensed. This situation may seem like a drawback but in reality often is not. Federal licensing of home day-care centers may involve the introduction of special toilets, low sinks, and designated areas for specific activities. These innovations must be paid for out of the pocket of the individual who is operating the program and thus raise a previously reasonable fee to one that may prove out of reach for many families.

There are many pluses for informal home day-care arrangements. First of all, they are relatively inexpensive ($40 to $70 per week, often with meals included). They also provide the kind of family and community experience that many child psychologists deem necessary for the development of healthy, well-adjusted children. The presence of other children, whether they are of similar or different ages, is very stimulating to babies. I used this kind of arrangement for my daughter from the time she was ten months old until she was almost two years. She had become too mobile for me to continue to take her to the studio, so I needed an alternative. The woman who operated this informal day-care home was a Dominican, named Olga, who had been in this country for about four years. Olga had been recommended to me by a friend, and she also took care of two other little girls. Though Olga was not highly educated, she had an extraordinarily good temperament and was gifted with children. She came from an exceptionally large family (her mother had had seventeen children) and so seemed to have a bottomless well of patience. She and Skye, my daughter, developed a loving relationship over the period of a year and a half my daughter stayed there. Though Spanish was the predominating language spoken, it did not seem to hinder Skye's development of English. Olga's daughter, Griselle, was an excellent student and fluent in both languages. When Griselle would return home from school, she would often sit with Skye and the other children and read stories or play imaginative games. It was as if Skye had two families. I seriously feel that both Olga and Griselle provided Skye with a valuable experience for that particular point in her development. Skye was exposed to another culture and another environment. She learned to be independent from her immediate family and learned that also other people could love her and provide for her. This independence, which she learned at an early age, is constantly evident to me.

When she goes to nursery school or music classes, children two and a half years old are literally clinging to their mother's legs begging not to be left, but Skye is giving me a hug and darting happily into the classroom, confident that I am returning.

I have chosen to discuss the licensed day-care center last because this particular child-care alternative seems to have no set standards. Even the privately run centers range from being highly inadequate, understaffed maintenance centers to being beautiful, loving support systems for the care of young children. A good infant and toddler care center will be expensive (from $80 to $140 per week), but it will often provide Pampers, nutritious meals, and a competent staff for this fee. Such centers, however, are few and are in such demand that there is often a waiting list of applicants. Due to the length of these waiting lists, it is recommended that you apply long before you give birth—perhaps as soon as you discover you are pregnant. These centers offer a high staff-to-child ratio—often about one adult for every two children. The play areas are creative and colorful—almost a child's paradise. Many of the toys available in these centers are designed to initiate and promote developmental skills. I am convinced that very few women at home alone could provide the wealth of stimulation that these particular centers give. Studies indicate that young children enrolled in these kinds of programs both speak and develop motor skills earlier and also interact better socially than children who have been raised in isolated environments. The main problem with these centers is that there are so few of them. You often have to know someone on the staff or an affiliate to get your child enrolled.

The long waiting lists and expense have forced most working mothers to seek alternative centers, but the problem alters drastically once your child reaches the age of two; there are many more adequate child-care and nursery programs available in this age category for families of almost all income levels. Before I discovered Olga, I had been looking for a licensed day-care program for Skye. The better child-care centers had extraordinarily long waiting lists, and there was no way Skye would be accepted into any of these programs in the immediate future. I had heard that the next best thing was to look for a child-care program affiliated with a religious organization. The problem I encountered there was that a majority of these programs would not accept children under the age of two. I did find one program that accepted children from the age of three months. It was supervised by an Episcopal priest and managed by a woman certified in early childhood education. But even with these criteria, it proved inadequate. Like many new mothers, I was ignorant of exactly what to look for in a child-care situation. First, though New York state, where I was a resident, requires the head of a child-care program to be certified, it sets no such standard for other staff members, and those staff members are often the ones who are most often in direct contact with your children. This particular center hired teenage girls to come in and take care of the children in the afternoon. These girls were untrained and often unsupervised. As a result, several of the infants in the program, including my daughter, broke out with a contagious disease called viral exanthem, which is a severe diaper rash caused by stale urine. The young girls were not changing the babies' diapers often enough and were not washing their hands between changings. When one baby acquired this rash, it was easily passed on to the next. This situation is not uncommon; women who have enrolled their children in a variety of substandard day-care programs have experienced it. Needless to say, I removed my daughter from this program right away.

Though it was a difficult lesson for me to learn, this situation illustrated the need for mothers to be able to evaluate day-care programs. Even though there are those few excellent infant and toddler care centers available, unless there is legislation insisting on an adequate standard for all child-care centers for children under the age of two, I personally feel that at present the informal family program may be more suitable for a child's needs than a substandard licensed child-care program if you are unable to get your child enrolled in an adequate one. My theory derives essentially from the influence of the environment in which child care takes place. When you invite someone into your own home, you are apt to treat them differently than if you greet them in your workplace. Your home is a personal reflection of yourself, while your workplace can be a reflection of a much larger body of people. The infant and toddler center that has superior resources and staff has a potential with which the less adequately financed center cannot possibly compete. However, if a family or an individual with similarly limited resources chooses to operate a child-care program from their home, they are motivated to put energy into it to compensate for the lack of finances; after all, it is their business, and they want it to be successful.

In addition, as I have said previously, the status of the American child-care worker must be improved for our child-care system to be improved. Early childhood education programs need to be expanded. When qualified men and women finish these programs, they should be able to receive funding and support from the government if they choose to establish centers of high quality. They should also be able to expect a decent salary for their efforts. Certified child-care workers should be recognized as a national resource and not viewed as providing a peripheral service. The bottom line seems to be society's and the government's recognition of organized child care as priority. A slogan coined by the Child & Parent Action Committee says, "It will be a great day when our centers have all the money they need and the navy has to hold a bake sale to buy a battleship."

Because so many centers are inadequate and because so many new mothers are unfamiliar with the criteria for evaluating care centers, I have included the following criteria as guidelines for determining the adequacy of a given center. These guidelines, as much of the advice I have offered in this book, are not absolutes; they merely serve to guide you to what your alternative may be.

Licensing

If in a given center there are more than six or seven children enrolled, federal and/or state licensing is almost always required. A large center run without the guidelines of the Federal Intragency Requiry, the organization that developed criteria for day-care centers, is not going to provide responsible care for your child. Federal licensing in general requires separate toilet and kitchen facilities for both staff and children. All children must be grouped separately in the following manner: one group for children up to twelve months old, one group for children ages one to two years, one group for children ages two to three years, and one group for children ages four to five years. All group divisions must have separate facilities and appropriate child/staff ratios commensurate with the developmental age of the group. Other federal stipulations will be discussed under the headings that follow. In general, the federal government makes the regulations for a day-care center's staff requirements and program structure, while the state regulates the building requirements of the day-care site. However, if the center provides for fewer than seven children, licensing may not be necessary even under the auspices of the federal government. Licensing in the latter circumstance may only hinder the operation of the facility, by imposing such requirements as the separation of children of diverse ages, which in a small operation may not be possible or practical.

Child-Staff Ratio

Ideally, in an infant and toddler care center, there should be no more than ten children in an individual play group. This group should be headed by a professional and supported by four adult assistants. This is a federal requirement in a licensed child-care center.

Hours

The question of hours depends upon your personal situation. If you are like most others of the working populace, it's likely you work forty hours per week, 9:00 A.M. to 5:00 P.M. each work day. If this is the case, a center that is open only during school hours, 9:00 A.M. to 3:00 P.M., will not serve your needs. Many centers, however, have now anticipated this need and are generally open from 8:00 A.M. to 6:00 P.M. General day-care hours are likely to be difficult for women who work odd hours (such as physicians, policewomen, and airline pilots). There is, unfortunately, no center serving all professions. However, if a second party, say your husband or baby-sitter, is elected to fill in for the hours you need to work and when the center is unavailable, you may still be able to adjust to a standard day-care situation.

Space

Do you feel the space is large enough for the allotted enrollment? Is it clean and brightly decorated, with a large partially carpeted indoor play area? Is there an outdoor play area as well? Large, clean, well-ventilated, well-heated space is absolutely necessary when caring for small children. The number of square feet required for each child in a day-care center varies in each state.

Safety

This is a particularly significant factor. The floors should be sanded, with no exposed nails, to avoid splinters and bruises. Windows, stairwells, and doorways should be equipped with safety guards. Storage equipment and other furniture should be sturdy with rounded edges—no rickety shelving or glass tables. Is the outdoor play equipment relatively safe? Are the toys carefully selected, with no small pieces that could be swallowed? Are cleaning and toiletry items kept safely out of reach?

Equipment

Though you may not be a child development expert, you can determine the quality of a facility's equipment. There should be an abundance of large blocks and balls, puzzles with large pieces, dolls, musical instruments, pull toys, books, training tricycles, and brightly colored plastic objects. It would be wise to see if these toys are in good working condition. Is there a sandbox, are there sufficient cribs and playpens for the infants, are there soft mats and blankets for the toddlers?

Program Organization

This is a vital factor in selecting an adequate center. My feeling is that children need more than custodial care. Studies have shown that infants as young as three months respond to being read stories. Exactly how is your child going to spend his or her day? What kind of structured activity is offered? Are there adequate rest and snack periods? Well-structured programs will often have a garden and small animals on the premises. Even from an extremely early age the introduction of plants and animals is very stimulating to young children. Are the children taken outside? Even a trip as mundane as going to the supermarket can be a learning experience for an infant or toddler. It is important for small children to be held and to be spoken to about every facet of life. Is there any effort made to teach children certain concepts, such as parts of the body or the names of animals or common objects? Most important, do you feel that the staff is conscientiously providing the kind of affection, information, and activities that you as a parent consider valuable?

Staff Training and Personality

There should be a full-time educational director at any facility providing for more than forty children. This is a federal regulation. His or her training should include doctoral or graduate-level work in early childhood education. This person should act only in a supervisory capacity and not be required to perform as a group teacher as well. All group heads should be certified as early childhood educators, and their assistants should be student teachers or experienced adults in early childhood education, although this is not absolutely necessary. More important than the staff's training, however, is the personalities of the people and their personal dedication to children. This factor, of course, is difficult to measure on any scale. More often than not your basic feeling about someone can be relied upon in determining whether or not a staff member is satisfactory.

Parent Participation

This may seem like an arbitrary point, but input from parents is often significant in determining the quality of the center. Is there a parent association? Are there frequent parent/teacher meetings to discuss your children? How much say do the parents have in the running of the center? Are the parents' suggestions taken seriously and used to improve the quality of the center? Such policies are crucial if you want to have input on how your child is cared for.

Miscellaneous

Though not absolutely necessary, the provision of hot meals, snacks, juice, milk, formula, and Pampers is often convenient and worth considering in the total evaluation of a center. The daily hauling back and forth of such items can be cumbersome and time-consuming. In general, a center should provide at least one hot meal and two nutritious snacks, such as cheese or apple slices (as opposed to pretzels or lollipops), if a child is there for an eight-hour period. Door-to-door transportation can also be found at some centers. It then becomes necessary to inspect the car or bus for appropriate car seats. Though not always available, transportation is an asset because it eliminates additional commuting time.

When evaluating care centers, try to visit at least three separate facilities before making a final choice. Assessments of cost and vicinity should also be taken into consideration but ideally should be placed lower on the evaluation scale than the child-staff ratio or program organization. A good center that may be slightly more expensive and farther away is certainly a better choice than a closer and less expensive but poorly organized center. Naturally, if a center is very inconveniently located or far over your budget limit it should not be considered in the first place.

The final question and perhaps the most emotionally charged issue concerning child care is "How is a child-care situation going to affect my child's relationship with his father and me? Will he still love us the same? Will he know that we are his parents?" One woman reports,

> *I just don't know how to feel. I was so uncomfortable when I heard her call Jenny (the baby-sitter) "Mommy." I wasn't sure if I wanted to share this relationship.*

I went through the same experience with my baby-sitter but somehow I didn't have the same ultimate reaction. Though initially I was confused about Skye calling Olga "Mommy," later I was comforted by that development. At that particular time I was working about fifty, sometimes sixty hours a week, seeing Skye only briefly during the week and on weekends. I considered the relationship that Olga and Skye developed a kind of security for me. To have your child love and trust another human being almost in the same way that she or he trusts you is, I feel, a relief. You can do what is important to you and know that your child is happy and well cared for. This feeling, of course, means that you give up some of your ego. You are not and are never going to be the only person in your child's life. Your child is learning a valuable skill in a day-care situation—that of loving and trusting a community of people other than just his immediate family. Research[13] over the past ten years has indicated again and again that it is the quality of the parent-child relationship, specifically of the mother-child relationship, that is far more significant than the actual amount of hours spent together. The most recent information indicates that the mother-child relationship of the mother who is a career woman and her children may actually be better than the relationship between the mothers who stay home with their children, since the time that the mothers with careers spend with their children is far more valuable to them because it is at a premium. There is absolutely no research to date that indicates that mothers who work outside the home have inadequate relationships with their children.

Relationships are built on consistency and intensity and not on specifically who gives a child a cookie at 3:00 p.m. Children are extremely flexible and intuitive. They will know instinctually that their primary relationships are with their families. The final criteria rest with you and your husband. If you can give warmth, compassion, and trust in the hours that you and your child spend together, you will be creating the relationship of love and security that fosters a strong parent-child relationship.

Integrating Your Lifestyle: The Marriage/Career/Family Balancing Act

Much of being a successful career woman and a successful mother at the same time is just plain logistics—where, when, and how to do things most efficiently. Though it may be a mundane issue in and of itself, the organization of your own and of your family's life is crucial to your effectiveness in the workplace and to your ability to function at home. The first thing you must do is establish priorities. You may have to accept the fact that the freedom you enjoyed before motherhood may no longer exist. Certain activities may have to be eliminated from your life, at least temporarily, for you to be able to maintain a realistic daily schedule.

When you have made the choice to return to work, sit down with your husband and map out your strategy on paper. Establish what household chores you will each take responsibility for, what your housekeeper will do, and what an older child may be able to do. There are certain chores that must be accomplished. Food must be purchased, clothing must be laundered, dishes must be washed, and the house should be kept clean. These kinds of "must do" chores should be considered before other, less pressing, chores, such as waxing the kitchen floor or scrubbing the bathtub. There are several methods by which a family can divide the household work. The first is awarding a specific chore to a specific person for a certain amount of time. For example, your husband will wash the dishes this week and you will do the marketing. Another way is dividing the chores by days. Your husband does the household chores on Monday, Wednesday, and Friday and you do them on Tuesday, Thursday, and Saturday, and you alternate on Sundays. If one parent is home significantly more than the other, it may be logical for him or her to accept a larger bulk of the household load, but this is largely a subjective decision. There may also be the need to eliminate some chores completely or to find someone else to do them. For instance, neither my husband nor I cook with any great regularity. I had thought this practice an unusual one, but on talking with other working mothers I found that many women give up cooking as soon as their child arrives. I am not offering this as a suggestion for everyone; it is certainly not practical for all, but it works for my husband and me. I am a vegetarian and my husband seldom eats meat except in restaurants, so the need to cook is not pressing. As alternatives, we eat easily prepared yet nutritious foods and also frequent restaurants. Skye enjoys the same simply prepared foods that we do and eats restaurant food as well. The second income I earn allows us to make this choice. I am not using our example to motivate anyone to stop cooking, but our situation does indicate that there are options available to anyone who can set aside previous habits and begin to explore alternatives. If you must do your own housekeeping, you and your husband can take a few tips from Heloise, the noted writer-columnist, who spent a lifetime trying to save time in the American household. New parents can rarely keep an immaculate home but you can attain neatness and a sense of order with the proper planning. The following housekeeping routine is a suggestion from Heloise and can be completed in less than two hours, leaving you with plenty of time for more important ventures.

When you and your husband get out of bed in the morning, the bed should be made immediately. Take all the dirty dishes, place them in the sink with detergent, and run hot water over them. You don't have to do the dishes right away—just let them soak. Now take two large shopping bags. Into one throw all the garbage that has accumulated in your house— tissues, diapers, newspapers, and so on. In the other bag place all the things that need to be put away—toys, books, clothing. Put the garbage bag in the kitchen and the "put-away" bag in the closet. The trick to this system is never to put or throw away an item individually; this takes too long and can make the early morning clean-up more drudgery than it is worth. Now take a paper towel and wet it with rubbing alcohol and go over the fixtures in the bathroom. Alcohol is an excellent disinfectant, is economical, and does a fairly decent cleaning job as well.

Now you or your husband can take a little rest and feed your baby. When your baby is satisfied, go into the kitchen and clean the dishes and empty the garbage. Go back to the closet, take out the "put-away" bag, and begin to sort. Put the dirty clothes in one pile and separate the remaining items according to the room in which they belong. Take each pile and put it in the appropriate room. If you need to do some laundry, gather all your soiled clothing and add it to the first pile. After you have started the washing machine go into each room and put away the items left.

Now your house is relatively clean, your bed is made, your dishes are done, your bathroom is sparkling, and your laundry is under way. Even if you don't get time to tackle those bigger projects today, you won't feel frustrated, because your house at least *looks* presentable.

In addition, before your baby has arrived, go through your house and do a thorough housecleaning. Give away to charity or to your friends those possessions that you have no use for. The less you have, the less there is to clean and the less clutter will be created. Before you purchase anything, ask yourself, "Will this make my life easier or more difficult?" If the answer is the latter, think twice about your purchase. Set up a specific area for your baby's things. This area can grow to become your child's play area, and having it will eventually keep blocks and toy trucks from filtering into your living room. These simple procedures will help you conserve your energy for the more vital tasks important to your own well-being.

When you and your husband have developed a tentative plan, review it weekly or even daily if need be. It is never going to be perfect and will need constant adjustments. There is a certain amount of flexibility required in all plans, for life is never consistent.

As I have indicated earlier, ongoing communication with your employer will be extremely important. Though letting him know the intimate facets of your personal life is never recommended, do let your employer know ahead of time if there is going to be any pressing family issue that you will need to attend to.

As for your time at home with your child, try to arrange a specific time each day to spend together. If may be as little as one hour per day that you can focus your energy totally on him. Even if your child cannot talk yet, it is important that you talk to him. You can play simple games, read stories, or sing. Whatever you do, allow your child to know that this is your special time together; don't chat on the phone, make business memos, or clean the sink when you want to focus your attention on him.

Your husband and you also need to be alone with each other. This means more than just staring at the television together in total exhaustion after you finally get the baby to sleep. Good long talks before you go to bed are a good method of communication, but arranging a date is even better. Try to go out together at least once a week. This can be an expensive proposition, considering current baby-sitting fees, but it can really give a boost to your relationship. Go to a movie or out to dinner, or just take a leisurely stroll together.

In the final analysis, the time you spend completely alone may actually be the most important thing for your emotional stability, yet it may be the most difficult to come by. Most parents are so immersed in just trying to be alone with each other that they forget the need for solitude. I strongly encourage each parent to find a special time to be alone at least once a week. This is a time in which you should not be doing housework or work-related projects; rather, it should be playtime or quiet time for yourself. This is actually quite simple to achieve if both parents agree to cooperate. One of you will babysit while the other "does his thing." This practice is especially effective when the two of you have been under pressure and there is no baby-sitter to help out. Rather than staying home and quibbling with each other or allowing your child to drive you crazy, one of you can take off and have a good long job in the park. These simple yet often unconsidered solutions are sometimes the best medicine for frazzled parents.

To conclude, parenting requires compromise. Some of these compromises may include career sacrifices on the part of both parents. Neither of you may be able to take as many out-of-town assignments or to go on prolonged business trips as you may have been able to do previously. You may have to make some social adjustments as well. You may not be able to attend all of the cocktail parties and gallery openings you want. However, compromises like these are often made by parents who feel that their roles as family members have priority over other aspects of life. Good parenting accompanied by career effectiveness can be accomplished with planning, support, and a loving commitment from both family partners.

=6=

"I HAVE A FAMILY"

The family, not the individual, is the real molecule of society, the key link in the social chain of being.
—Robert Nisbet, *Twilight of Authority*

It is a very different feeling to be living in "threes" than to be living in "twos." Though there are many couples who consider themselves a family, the word "family" in Western society conjures up a slightly different picture. A family includes children. Bride and groom, husband and wife is one concept, but being mother and father is quite another. If there is one single thing you can expect from new parenthood, it is change. Unlike previous generations, our generation can more easily plan a family, but no matter how well-planned a child is, there will be times filled with parental anxiety and doubt when we may feel literally terrified of the small child and of our parental roles. One new mother has expressed her apprehension in this way:

Some days I just feel like pulling the blanket over my head. I panic. I just cannot get up and run to the market for a quart of orange juice anymore. I have to prepare for even the simplest excursion.

A new father speaks of his fears:

> *I don't know. I may sound sexist, but Caroline—she's had all the training. She took care of her younger sisters and baby-sat for other kids. No one ever told me anything about babies, and I'm afraid. I simply don't know what to do.*

Inadequacy, responsibility—these are the feelings of new parenthood. And perhaps these fears are heightened by the changing role of the family in society. The family in which Mom stays home and Dad goes to work is being outmoded. Only 34 percent of the families in this country fit this pattern. More than half of the families in this country have two parent wage earners. These new families have in essence become pioneering families, marking out new paths to emotional security, independence, and happiness.

Choosing to become parents is a difficult decision. You may see the mistakes of your own parents or the state of the world and shake your head and say, "No, never." But again, you may feel that if you do not have children, you may miss an important experience.

You may also have a more personal wish to become a parent. You may have had a wonderful family experience and want to relive that with a child of your own. Or you may look at your spouse and think that you will give each other the present of yourself in a new human being. But whatever the reason, the choice to have a child is a significant life decision. It is a rite of passage, so to speak, redefining ourselves and our lives in terms of another person.

During the course of pregnancy, you may be so wrapped up in your own anticipation that you may neglect to consider other realities. Many parents return from the hospital before they have considered making the appropriate adjustments for parenthood. Though it is never too late to make arrangements, when you return from the hospital you may be so overwhelmed by the childbirth experience that you may not be able to think clearly. You and your spouse may wind up staring at each other, wondering what wizardry it will take to raise the child. You may wonder why you don't all of a sudden *feel* like a parent. After all, you may think, isn't parenting instinctual?

Unfortunately, parenting is not an innate ability. In human beings it is learned behavior. And, like playing the piano or riding a bicycle, which is also learned behavior, parenting takes practice. Your first child will often be examined, as if under a magnifying glass, for responses; you seem to be asking him, "Hey, kid, how am I doing?" Everyone wants to be a good parent, to do the right thing.

However, we often have such high expectations of ourselves as parents that we are bound to fail. New infants are totally demanding and rarely predictable. The first few months we have to reorganize our lives completely, and we may resent having to do so. There are going to be real obstacles to maintaining your family balance. A family cannot be run like a business; you may not be able to see profits or to break even for a long time. Solutions may lie in committing yourselves totally to shared parenthood and in accepting that the confusion of the first few months of parenting is absolutely normal and not directly reflective of your parenting skills.

In this chapter I will try to provide you with a script—a running dialogue of what may happen emotionally during your first year of parenting. I will describe methods of shared parenting that have worked for me. And I have also included a section on fathering, a topic that is often neglected. I will also discuss the parents' love relationship—how that will change as a result of parenthood and how you can cope with that change. Last, I will discuss how you can develop a good relationship with your baby.

Parenting is not merely an obligation. Parenting does tend to fill a special need in most of us who choose that role. Parenting can expose our weaknesses, but it also magnifies our strengths. When I see my daughter standing in front of the mirror with outstretched arms, singing "Jimmy, Crack Corn," I think to myself, what a confident child she is; she seems to like herself so much. I must be doing a pretty good job. And it gives me confidence.

Moments like these, though few, can make up for the hours of your baby's crying, the endless pools of spilled apple juice, the sleepless nights you've spent, and the sometimes scrambled hours of work when all that parenting seems to do is get in the way of your personal goals. Most important, as parents you must try to take care of each other during this time, as well as taking care of your baby. Remember, you may be taking care of each other a long time after your baby is gone and is having babies of his own.

"The Man I Love": Your Husband

As women are trying to pull themselves together and make their mark in the outside world, some men are eagerly trying to crawl back into their homes and be recognized as significant there. As one father confides,

> *I never felt that my father really cared about my sister and me. He might have meant well but he never tried to be with us. I don't want to be like that. I want my son to know that I can do more than just pay the bills and give spankings.*

The sensitive man has emerged from the rubble of the feminist movement and he wants to be counted. If a woman can have the baby blues, then a man can have the husband blues. *Family Health*[1] magazine coined the term "husband blues" in 1977 in a discussion of "feelings to experience and emotional changes to be aware of during and after pregnancy" in new fathers. Most men undergo an emotional change when they first become fathers. Some new fathers, like new mothers, have a violent reaction to the birth of their children—so much so that it affects their ability to function on a variety of levels. There are documented cases of postpartum depression in men severe enough to warrant psychiatric intervention. However, these cases—though significant—are not representative of most new fathers.

Men are often accused of envy or of being unsupportive of their wives during postpartum recovery. However, in many instances the father is not jealous of his baby or his wife specifically but feels he is being left out. It is his baby, too, but all that society expects of him is to make a decent salary and to be the "head" of the family.

As sexist as our society is in awarding total parental responsibility to the woman, it is just as sexist in taking this responsibility away from the man. Psychologists, social workers, childcare workers, and pediatricians are much more comfortable discussing children in relation to their mothers than in relation to their fathers. They expect fathers to be busy in the office; they think that fathers don't want to hear about stomachaches, teething, or diarrhea. But many fathers want to share parenting and often feel that basic social structures are hindering them from doing so.

Anthropologists have long established that men, in general, have always struggled to find compensation for the fact that the female sex is able to give birth and that males can offer society no genuine equivalent. There are numerous theories about male-oriented activities such as hunting, rites of initiation into manhood, and even misogyny, which explain that these activities demonstrate man's need to compensate for the biological fact that he can never give birth. However, none of these theories have provided the apparent solution to this problem. If men want to have the same status as women as far as parenting is concerned, they need to be involved totally in the parenting process.

As women need to fulfill themselves as people, so do men. But women can also be at fault in shared parenting situations. Even though a woman may value her career in the same manner that her husband values his, she may still resent her husband's intrusion in the nursery. She may consider certain tasks maternal and not welcome her husband's interest. One woman describes her feelings in this way:

> I feel that John is too rough with the baby. He throws him up in the air and wrestles with him. Because of my own upbringing, I sometimes feel uneasy about this, yet Joey [her son] loves it and loves his father. I guess in order to foster this shared parenting, I just have to step back and allow my husband and my child to develop their own relationship on their own terms.

Stories such as this are numerous and include complaints about the way a father may dress his child, or how he may allow his daughter to get too dirty or his son to climb too high. Individual images of parenting are going to conflict in the best of marriages. And even if you both have the same essential goals, your methods of arriving at these goals are often going to be different and reflect your own personal family experiences. There will be instances in which both you and your husband will have to compromise and perhaps review some of your parenting expectations.

Another interesting, though not surprising, phenomenon is that many new mothers who feel threatened by their husbands' insistence on sharing parental responsibility will begin to belittle, unjustly and often unconsciously, their husband's efforts. One new father remarks:

> Whenever I take a day off to be with Alysse, my wife will call me twelve times a day from her office. It is as if she is terrified that I will forget where the Baby Magic is or forget to feed her. I'm an adult and I surely can find my way around my own house.

Another new mother states:

I know Dan can handle things at home, but somehow I just get nervous whenever he's at home with the baby and I'm at work. I get preoccupied thinking that he won't know what time to start dinner or give Elana her bath.

Why are some women so uncomfortable with this new sensitive man? Perhaps those cartoons of the hapless husband, apron around his waist, smoking a cigar, and making mincemeat of the household have affected some women more than they would like to admit. Remember the "Dick Van Dyke Show"? In one episode, Laura, Rob's wife, went back to work in television as a dancer. Rob had to come home from work at night to keep house and take care of his son, Richie. Because Rob was so inept at household duties, he and Richie ended up eating bananas every night for dinner. Of course, Laura eventually gave up her dancing job. Rob was presented as inept at homemaking, and Laura was presented as equally inept at maintaining an outside job. Almost every pre-1965 television situation comedy had a segment similar to the one just described. It was automatically assumed that, if a wife went to work, the husband would never be able to cope with making his family's dinner.

Society has assumed that most men, with the exception of the great chefs of the world and a few "gentlemen's gentlemen," are not able to cook, do the laundry, and, most of all, handle the demands of a newborn child. But many men can and want to do those tasks. If wives are afraid to allow their husbands' full participation in parenting, it may be due to the fact that many women still do not have careers as prestigious as their husbands' and, in order to balance the scales more, may try to be better housekeepers and parents than their husbands.

Women, as well as men, have to rethink seriously traditional sex stereotypes. Infants and small children need to interact with men as much as they do with women. As important as it is for a child to see his mother independent and secure, he also needs to see his father as a warm, accessible person.

Joseph Pleck, researcher and author of *Men and Masculinity*, believes that men bond emotionally with their newborn infants in very much the same way that women do. His theory is heavily supported by the psychologists Greenberg and Morris, who have conducted extensive studies on father and child relations:

> Fathers of newborns showed engrossment in their infants, a sense of bonding, absorption, and preoccupation in their child, which Greenberg and Morris interpreted as innate potential in fathers which was released by exposure to the infant . . . they were strongly attached to their infants and focused their attention on him or her, they could distinguish their child's cry from others', and . . . they felt extreme elation and increased self-esteem because of their child.[2]

Men are not often taught to give in this society. When they do give, they are often conditioned to expect something in return. Parenting may be the only opportunity that the average man has to experience the joy of total giving. Harry Finkelstein Keshel, codirector of the Brandeis University fathering study, confirms this theory:

> When you have a man willing to give because someone needs you to give or they'll die or won't develop—that's a rare experience and it's in parenting that men can have that experience.[3]

As I have described in a previous chapter, paternal instincts have been studied in many cultures and also in the animal world. There is a term, "couvade," which both anthropologists and psychologists have used to describe the dramatic sympathetic birthing experience of the husbands of pregnant women in certain cultures. During couvade a husband will lie next to his wife, contorting his body in an effort to mimic his wife's labor. Later, the husband will develop postpartum recovery symptoms, such as weeping and extreme sadness. In addition, there are many valid and intensive studies to indicate that a man can, under given conditions, be as good and loving a parent as any woman.

But what about the man who doesn't volunteer, who doesn't seem interested, and who leaves you stranded to juggle a new baby, a job, and a household? Such a situation may seem like a "cop-out," but it may not be entirely the man's fault. Without a strong "masculinist" movement, with men out there waving banners and demanding equal time for family intimacy, your husband's attitude very well may be "I was in the delivery room with you, wasn't I? What else do you want?" Many new fathers as well as new mothers do not fully understand the concept of shared parenting. An ideal shared parenting situation is one where careers, the housework, and parenting are divided equally, straight down the middle. This ideal, however, like other ideals, is rarely the reality. The average father, even if he works in his home or, because of a more flexible work schedule, is home more than his wife is, does not contribute significantly to household work or to actual child care. In the book *Child Development and Behavior*,[4] it is stated that in the United States, men contribute roughly about 1.6 hours combined housework and child care per day, with only about 12 minutes of that time used for primary child care. Another study[5] reviewed in the same book concludes that the average father spends exactly 38 seconds a day with his infant. The most time any man devoted to his newborn in this particular study was 10 minutes, 26 seconds per day. With such statistics, it is not surprising that 50 percent of preschool children interviewed for another study[6] said that they preferred television to the companionship of their fathers. With such established patterns and the fact that there are so few fathering support groups, it may be solely up to you to make parenting available to your husband.

This may be difficult, for you will be reversing some long-held sex stereotypes in the process. Boys, traditionally, are not taught to admire a man who possesses parenting skills. Children's stories, though they have had their share of Cinderellas, have always had a fair number of more realistic heroines. Jo in *Little Women*, Nancy Drew, Pippi Longstocking, and even Wonder Woman are all examples of female characters who are vital and exciting. While girls are often given masculine characters to emulate, boys are rarely given examples of nurturing males. As a result, men rarely associate nurturing with masculinity. Because of confusion about their new life roles, new fathers can often become angry and bitter over their wives' needs and feelings of inadequacy during postpartum recovery. Many husbands in reaction to their feelings of inadequacy may actually try to avoid their wives altogether. Speaking of her husband, one woman has said,

> *He never stays home anymore. He comes home to eat and then leaves for the racquet club. He can't stand the disarray or the exhausting pressure of our baby.*

Situations like the previous one, although not uncommon, are extreme and may represent an ambivalence toward parenting as well as other unresolved marital or personal conflicts. Having a child thrust into the center of your life can heighten feelings previously undealt with. But sometimes, because of the emotional intensity of postpartum recovery, couples may be forced into resolution. The same woman who previously describes her husband's hostility later relates:

> *I decided, after about two months of this intolerable situation, that I was going away to my sister's for the weekend and I wasn't taking the baby. When I returned the house was a mess and he was exhausted. He deeply apologized. He had been angry because he thought I wasn't taking our new responsibility as seriously as he was. He was working hard. The disorder at home and the baby always crying—that just seemed to be telling him that I didn't care.*

As there is open resistance to new mothers in the workplace, there is often resistance to the man who wants to make an equal contribution at home. Though employers, as a rule, have preferred the family man as an employee rather than the swinging bachelor, they don't often welcome his family concerns if they intrude upon his work. The career mother, on the other hand, though she is often discriminated against for this very attitude, is almost expected to have divided loyalties. After all, she is a mother. She is supposed to be concerned. But the man who leaves his office once too often to make an early pickup at the babysitter's is often, at best, seen by his colleagues as confused about his "real" priorities or, at worst, as eccentric. As the workplace must change so that women can achieve in the business and political spheres, so it must also change to allow men to experience childrearing fully. And the best time to begin fathering is right at the beginning. Emotionally, a child's personality is pretty well set before he enters kindergarten. By the time a child reaches the age of nine or ten and is thought by his father to be a good companion on a fishing trip, it is often too late for that father to have any intrinsic effect on that child's development.

Fathering can have its lonely moments as well. Often, if a father takes a child to the park for example, he'll find that the mothers there ignore him. He often has no cohorts. As one father explains:

> *Sometimes I feel uncomfortable. The women I meet in the playground are accommodating. But they certainly don't know what it is like to be the lone father. I feel like a pioneer. Where are all of the fathers, anyway?*

Even though shared parenting can have its difficult moments for fathers, most of those who choose to share in their wives' postpartum experience feel that, as a result, their self-image changes significantly and that their life goals achieve a new balance. One man confides:

> *I'm not so crazy at work anymore. Since my wife is earning a good salary, too, I don't have to make as much*

money as I thought I'd have to with a new baby. When five P.M. comes, I'm out of the office and going home to take Joshua to the park. I look forward to that. It makes more sense to me to be putting my energy into another human being rather than into some intangible account.

When a father has the equal or even partial financial support of his wife, it can relieve much of the economic stress that many fathers feel at the birth of a child. Shared parenting gives a father a new identity, which stems from more than just his bread-earning power; it stems from being treated as a caring person and being loved and respected for that identity. He becomes familiar with the spilled milk on the floor, the strawberry jam on the walls, and the endless parade of toys in the hallways. A father who shares parenting is no longer viewed by his children as the traditional austere disciplinarian, the individual who was most often noted for his absence in family affairs rather than his participation. Children will come to see their fathers as being truly committed to their lives and not as just the weekend providers of entertainment or as Little League coaches; both parents will take equal responsibility for the joys and woes of modern parenting.

"WILL WE EVER MAKE LOVE AGAIN?" SEX AND PARENTING

Aside from the fact that many gynecologists advise sexual abstention during the first six weeks of the postpartum period, as a precaution against pelvic infection, sexual intimacy during the postpartum year can become a psychological battlefield, once the sex act is medically allowed again. Perhaps worry about sex and parenting arises from the fact that in American culture we rarely equate sexual coupling with conceiving a child. Even though children are the biological result of sexual intercourse, sexual intimacy is not always seen as a prelude to the family, except by a few religious groups. When we, as adults, embark upon a new sexual relationship, we rarely envision a couple of kids at the foot of our beds on Sunday morning. Sex, in its romantic sense, does not include children.

Though not much is known about early man's sexual behavior, many anthropologists support the theory that much of our sexual behavior is the result of parenting behavior. Long ago, in the depths of the forest, when primitive man lived more by instinct, he did not kiss or caress his partner, nor did she him. They copulated without paying much attention to each other. Later, as parents, primitive people began to respond to the clinging behavior of their infants with hand stroking and the motion of placing their lips upon their infants' heads. Gradually, these gestures were transformed into the foreplay that often accompanies sexual intercourse. This theory is heavily supported by the contemporary behavior of many sexual couples; though we may be strong, independent adults in the outside world, we often behave as children do when we are with our lovers. The kind of behavior that I am referring to is not to be confused with pathological behavior, in which one searches for a parent figure rather than an equal when choosing a sexual partner. What I am referring to is the holding, the caressing, and the soft voices that lovers often use and that mimic the behavior of parent and child. Both men and women recognize this behavior as comforting and often initiative of enjoyable sexual relations. The intimacy that parenting requires can often strengthen the intimacy of a marriage. However, adults seldom notice this correlation. The baby who often remains in the bedroom during the early months of the postpartum period is often seen as a chaperone. As one mother has said:

> I think that he was born with a radar device that tells him when we are making love. Every time we begin, he awakens, howling to be fed and changed and soothed.

No one welcomes the interruption of their lovemaking. But the reality is that infants do awaken continually during the night and demand attention. When new parents try to ignore the shrieking, the situation seems to get worse. It is like making love with the television blasting or with construction workers hammering outside your window. Moreover, there will be evenings when feeding your child and taking care of it will leave you exhausted, with no time or energy for making love. So what can you do? During these early months, when your baby requires continual nocturnal attention, there may be little you can do except perhaps not expect too much. Other cultures accept the early postpartum period as a time of sexual abstention. Couples may not even sleep in the same bed. The mother may take the baby for half of the night and then give him to her husband for the remainder. If the baby awakens to be nursed while he is in his father's care, the father will simply bring the baby to his mother to be fed, wait until the baby is finished, and then take him back to bed with him. If the infant awakens for reasons other than to nurse, the father is responsible. In this manner, both parents are able to receive a reasonable amount of sleep. Though I am not suggesting sexual abstention as a rule, if you can realize that at least temporarily your sexual activity may be curtailed, you may be able to cope better. The other suggestion that is often offered as a solution to this problem is taking a brief vacation without the baby during the first few months. A weekend alone together, with nothing to do but stay in bed and make love, is often the best solution for new parents hungry for their own relationship.

There is also the fatigue factor at play during the early months. Both parents may simply be too exhausted from the overwhelming demands of career and parenting to want to make love. All you may want is a good night's sleep. This feeling can be acceptable. Neither partner should feel pressured into having sexual relations when he or she is fatigued or simply not in the mood. However, if this fatigue or lack of interest in sex continues for a relatively long period, it may be indicative of other feelings. Perhaps you are hostile toward your spouse because, in a sense, he or she has caused you to become a parent. Without your sexual relationship, you could be sleeping through the night. Deliberately withdrawing sex from your partner is often used as a weapon. If this happens, you could need some special counseling or simply a heart-to-heart talk with your spouse.

The fatigue that accompanies the postpartum period often acts as a blanket for feelings. You may simply need to make time for sex. With all the preparations you have made for other aspects of your life during the postpartum period, the pleasure of each other is often overlooked. Instead of going out for your ritual dinner and movie on Saturday night, arrange to have a sitter take care of your baby at his or her home. Then you can have time for each other at home. If you can afford it, rent a hotel room for the afternoon and take some time off from work and meet each other. This may sound rather odd—two married people running around as if they are conducting an illicit affair—but, in fact, anything you can do to foster your love relationship should be considered. You deserve a chance for romantic play.

As I have mentioned in previous sections good communication with your spouse is crucial. Good conversation makes for a good love relationship. Talking is absolutely necessary if you expect your marriage to work. Each day steal a few moments to be truly with each other. Don't talk about the baby. Don't talk about your job. You cannot automatically, on Friday night, turn on your romantic self and expect your relationship to be perfect. Love is a continuum. It may rise and fall, but it must always be there.

The last but certainly not the least significant issue regarding sex and parenting is that your children will most likely learn their sexual attitudes from you. Many of us grew up in a generation in which the idea that our parents were making love in the next room while we were asleep was totally alien to us. Today, we may not want to pass on to our own children the notion that the sex act is taboo or mildly subversive. A number of psychologists now believe that, biologically, sexuality begins *in utero.* Infants a day old can respond physically to sexual stimuli. But in order for children to appreciate their psychological sexual identities, they need cues from their parents.

Although I don't believe in the exploitation of the human body, I do feel that, in order to foster sexual identities in our children better, the whole concept of family nudity in this culture needs to be seriously reviewed. In one Cleveland study,[7] more than half of the parents interviewed felt that it was wrong for children to see their parents naked. Nudity in the home is thought to promote incest or perversion. Personally, I feel that the absence of nudity promotes deviant behavior. I am certainly not suggesting that everyone strip off clothing and run around the house naked, but there is no reason for a small child not to see you while you are taking a bath or going to the toilet. Many pediatricians now condone communal showering and bathing as a prelude to a child's healthy sexual image. Exposure of the human body also has its practicality; a young child who sees his parents using the toilet is more prone to adopt this behavior for himself. A recent study[8] has revealed that teenage girls who had never seen their fathers' or brothers' penises were often terrified of seeing a naked man, as if the penis was a frightening object. A child needs to see from a very early age that there are two sexes and that there are explicit sexual differences. Of course, if you are extremely uncomfortable being nude in your child's presence, it may be best not to be nude, as you may pass on your uncomfortable feelings to your child rather than the positive sexual image you might want to foster. But, in general, body image is extremely important to self development, and children need to think of their bodies as acceptable.

Should children see their parents making love? This is a topic over which there is controversy. In my opinion, if a child happens to see his parents engaging in sexual intercourse, that in and of itself is not psychologically damaging. However, if a child is allowed by his parents to view the sexual act at his own whim, I feel that such permissiveness takes sexual intercourse out of its social context. Sexual intercourse is a private act. It is not a "bad thing," but we may not want other people around during it. If your toddler accidentally awakens from his nap and sees you engaging in sexual intercourse, it is important for you to remain calm and not get alarmed or angry. Your child could be frightened by the movement or sounds of the sex act and may need to be reassured. A child does not understand the nature of sexual coupling until preadolescence. However, you can explain to him that Mommy and Daddy love each other very much and, because they do, they like to hold and hug each other. This very simple information is often all a toddler needs or can understand. If he does not seem upset, it may simply be that he hasn't noticed anything peculiar. If you regard his intrusion casually, then so will he.

To reiterate from Chapter One, there are medical reasons for abstention from sexual intercourse during the early postpartum period. The vaginal barrel needs to remain clear to prevent pelvic infection, and if you have had an episiotomy, your stitches will need to heal. However, there is no reason for you and your husband to avoid other forms of sexual activity. Sexuality is an extremely vital part of our lives, and in order for it to be fully realized we need to have maturity, patience, and respect. Postpartum recovery is a difficult time for all new parents, and your love and desire for each other must often be tempered by understanding that your life situation has changed. You will make love again, and hopefully your lovemaking will be strengthened and heightened by your new roles as parents.

"Mommy and Daddy": Being Parents

I can't tell you how to become good parents, at least not in the relatively short span of this section. Parenting and parenting skills are the subject matter of many books. What I can give you here is an idea of what it feels like to be a parent, some fundamental parental guidelines, and perhaps a few suggestions on how to keep from going crazy. Being a parent is often compared to being a circus performer. At six P.M. the average family situation can be something like the following, in the words of one working mother:

Bob is making a salad and Jenny is sitting in her high chair playing with a spoon and drinking apple juice from her bottle. The phone rings. It's my mother. She wants to know how things are going. I tell her things are fine. Just then Jenny drops her bottle, whose cap is loose, spilling apple juice onto the floor and into my shoe. Bob heads to mop the juice up and knocks the salad bowl over in the process. Jenny is now banging with her spoon, on her metal high-chair tray. I tell my mother that due to the spoon banging, I cannot hear and will have to call her back. I climb over the juice and the salad with my one soaked shoe and futilely try to assist Bob in collecting the remnants of our dinner. Jenny is screaming now. She wants her puréed vegetables and tapioca pudding. I stop cleaning the floor, pick her up, and go through the cabinets selecting Beechnut jars. Jenny is straddling my hip now. She refuses to allow me to put her down. Somehow, she thinks that if I put her down, she won't eat. My husband is still on the floor cleaning the mess and I am performing the maneuvers of an octopus, holding Jenny with one arm and heating the baby food with the other. The salad is off the floor now, along with the spilled juice. Bob begins to prepare another salad. I gather Jenny and her dinner in my arms, seat her in her chair, and begin to feed her. Bob sets my salad in front of me, along with a glass of club soda. Jenny doesn't want her baby food anymore. She wants my salad. She is slopping her own meal everywhere to punctuate her disdain. I am angry now. There is puréed something or another in my salad. I ask Bob to finish feeding Jenny. I sit down, sipping my club soda. I ask myself, "What are we doing wrong?"

There is an early moment in parenting with which many parents can identify. It usually occurs within the first week of delivery. This feeling tends to enter like a phantom, slowly and without notice. Initially, you may be distracted by the whirlwind of well-wishers come to visit the new parents and the new baby, and then one morning you face the reality. You have a totally helpless infant that is totally dependent upon you for everything. I don't think there is any equivalent life experience, with perhaps the exception of caring for an ailing parent or sibling, in which we must take on such great responsibility. And most of us do not enter parenting with this kind of experience. No matter how many friends you may have who have children or how intimate your own family relations may have been, the truth of family life never quite affects you the same way as when you have children of your own.

I feel that there are two major myths concerning parenting that are especially damaging to the parenting image we may hold of ourselves. The first is that by virtue of becoming a parent you are an adult, fully mature, in no further need of growing. As Gail Sheehy states in her book, *Passages*,[9] adults never stop developing. Also, how you feel about parenting may be determined by the stage of adult development in which you become a parent. I feel that a woman who has established her career and as a result has become secure, will have a far different view of parenting than a young girl who has had no exposure to the outside world. However, because of the myth about adulthood that I have mentioned, many parents feel embarrassed by their own needy feelings. Parents are simply human beings. The birth of a child and the adjustment it involves leave many parents overwhelmed and in need of support from each other and from other parents.

The second myth is that parenting is instinctual. It is not. It is learned behavior that requires the same dedication and interest involved in learning any other skill.

Early parenting images have been described to me in many ways:

It's like living in a tunnel. You can't see all around you anymore—only straight ahead and straight behind!

It's like dancing to strange music that you've never heard before and don't particularly like. After a while, though, you get used to it.

Gordon Hanson, in his fascinating paper "Learned Parenthood: Tending Raw Eggs,"[10] writes that one high-school teacher related the experience of early parenthood by making her students carry a raw egg with them wherever they went.

My image of my own early experiences in parenting was that of a jigsaw puzzle that never got finished. I saw my life in many tiny fragments, and I had to look carefully for the correct interlocking pieces. Sometimes I would find a piece that would appear to link to another and I would meticulously hammer away trying to make the prospective piece fit. It was all a matter of searching and discarding, searching and discarding, until I found something that worked. I often felt that my puzzle had been purchased without all the necessary pieces to complete my picture. But I soon realized this particular life puzzle wasn't meant to be completed. Every day I would just add another piece.

Parents are often worried about what kind of parents they are going to be. Will they make the same mistakes their parents did? How do they know they are doing the right things? Before you decide what kind of parent you are going to be, you have to determine what kind of person you are. What would you like your child to know, to feel? These are very significant questions to ask yourself even at the earliest point in your child's development. There is a wealth of evidence to support the theory that a child's personality is formed by the time he or she is two years old, and how you relate to your child will affect his development considerably.

Though my husband's and my feelings concerning parenting skills are our own, I feel that they do represent a fair cross section of psychological and social theories regarding parenting today. You, of course, will have to define your own parenting beliefs. We believe in a balance of freedom and discipline. Since small children do not understand the word "no" until they are well over a year old, and since we wanted our child to have the freedom of lots of space, we redecorated our apartment. We put all of our potentially dangerous and delicate items out of reach and allowed Skye a certain amount of physical independence. I knew, having been trained as a movement therapist, that a child's sensory development is initiated and enhanced by his relationship to his immediate environment.

Along with allowing this physical freedom, my husband and I felt we needed to establish a few rules as well. For instance, except in extreme circumstances, such as having a nightmare or feeling sick, Skye was not permitted to sleep with us. She was allowed to lie in bed with us for a short time if she chose to, but we then expected her to return to her crib. We insisted on this rule after her first months of nursing had concluded, because both my husband, Randy, and I felt that a child should sleep in his own bed to learn self-sufficiency. Many parents may disagree—perhaps considering this cruel— but we strongly felt that even a young child needed to see a clear line between his own life and his parents' life.

We instituted a code of discipline early on. If Skye went near a dangerous object, such as a hot stove or the bathtub, after we had repeatedly warned her against doing this, we would slap her hand. Though we don't believe in corporal punishment as a rule, we felt that in cases where injury was imminent, the slap on the hand was certainly better than the burn or the bump on the head she might have incurred. I must add that we didn't immediately slap her hand upon her approaching the object. We would first bark a sharp no; then, if she persisted, we moved her from the dangerous area. If, however, she continued to endanger herself, we used the slap as a form of negative reinforcement. Also, in order to keep her from focusing her attention on these intriguing no-nos, we tried to absorb her in activities which we felt would be more interesting than the forbidden actions.

We also feel, as parents, that the concept of good versus bad is not necessarily productive. Though there are some actions which are wrong in any context, we feel that most actions are simply appropriate or inappropriate. For example, if Skye was seated happily banging her drum while I was idly leafing through a magazine, I would consider her drum playing appropriate behavior. However, if she chose to bang that same drum while I was at my desk writing, I would no longer consider that action appropriate. If her action was deemed inappropriate, she would be offered a substitute activity or be removed to another corner of the apartment where her action would not be disturbing. But we would never tell her that she was "bad" simply because she had been playing the drum.

Anger was another issue we dealt with. Many parents feel uncomfortable about displaying anger to their children, especially anger that may be specifically directed at them. We feel, however, that anger, as long as it does not result in physical abuse, is a valid emotion. If we become angry, we let Skye know it. Children also become angry, and parents have to find room for their children's anger, too. We even felt that if we became angry over one of Skye's actions that was completely innocent, she would still be able to learn a valuable lesson from this anger. In life, people do become angry over insignificant issues as well as vital ones. If this happened, we would always apologize to her once we realized that our anger had been unwarranted. Essentially, we believe that the repression of real anger is needed only in rare circumstances. Many times Randy or I would become angry at something that had nothing to do with Skye. We, as a family, have learned to leave room for the personal anger of another. When I am angry, I can be pretty dramatic! Skye will wait until I calm down and then come over to me and say, "Finished now, Mommy?" and purse her lips for a kiss. Children can learn to live with their parents' emotions, provided these emotions are genuine and provided that the children are allowed the same emotional privileges that their parents have.

Should you give your child everything he wants? Can you spoil him? A child under three months old is incapable of being spoiled. To become spoiled, you need to have some identification with the outside world. The newborn infant hasn't developed that sense. Around the age of twelve weeks, an infant has learned that crying gets a response and will cry for more reasons than just essential biological needs such as being hungry or being uncomfortable and wanting to be changed. He begins to cry to be held or to be looked at. You should respond to these cries also, because in this manner you set the precedent for your primary relationship with your child. At around six months, a child will begin to cry because he wants a particular object, and he will often cry until he gets what he wants. Sometimes what he wants will be compatible with your wishes, other times it will not. Personally, Randy and I didn't feel that a child over six months should be given everything that he or she wants. Some parents, often due to exhaustion, will give in to a screaming child and as a result only end up teaching that child one thing, "If I scream loud and long enough, I will get what I want." You can observe countless examples of this practice with slightly older children in supermarkets. These children begin their slow whine for chocolate and fruit punch at the market's threshold. The parents will retort with an endless repetition of nos. Finally, the parents, in an effort to shut the kid up, surrender and buy the bar of chocolate and the carton of punch. These parents have rewarded inappropriate behavior. My husband and I wanted to nip this behavior in the bud. Whenever Skye would shriek for something, we would ignore her and wait until she stopped. When she stopped crying, she would be rewarded with the wanted object if we considered that object appropriate. If what she wanted was not appropriate, we offered her a substitute. What she learned here was that screaming, which is rarely acceptable behavior, would not be rewarded. (*Note:* This practice was never used in response to essential functions. If she cried because she was hungry or otherwise uncomfortable, we always attended to those needs.) Even today, both Randy and I insist that Skye make requests in an acceptable manner. If she shrieks for her apple juice, she does not receive it until she calms down. We also still use substitutes, now that she's four years old. Skye would probably eat ice cream all day if we allowed it. However, when she asks for ice cream at an inappropriate time, we offer yogurt instead. This practice has worked very well.

The final concept regarding parenting skills that I wish to discuss is that of sex stereotypes. I discussed this topic at some length in Chapter Five. Children should, of course, know whether they are male or female, and they will normally acquire this concept at or around the age of two. However, I feel that the concept of gender must be arrived at without the intrusion of traditional sex stereotypes. Letty Cottin Pogrebin, in her commendable book *Growing Up Free*, discusses this subject with great clarity and sensitivity. The choice of toys and clothing should be careful and specific from a very early age. Girls should be given a variety of playthings, including the stereotyped male trucks and construction toys, and boys should have dolls and dishes, among their other toys, in their toy box to avoid stereotypes. Some may ask, "Doesn't this practice encourage homosexuality?" This is often the argument against reversing or breaking down traditional stereotypes. Though no one as yet knows the true causes of homosexuality, the evidence available supports the theory that it is the presence of strong stereotypes that may eventually lead to homosexuality and not the reverse. This is not to say that Susie should never wear ruffles. As long as both your son and daughter are encouraged to explore and not blindly accept the traditional roles, you can be sure you are promoting the correct attitudes toward sexual identity.

With all my discussion of the practicalities of shared parenting, you may be wondering about its emotional aspects. What are the emotional components of shared parenthood?

There needs to be love between the parents and the child. This love transcends just caring for your child in a rudimentary fashion. It involves thinking and being concerned about your child even when you are not with her or him.

The second element is time. Though the concept of quality time cannot be dismissed, each parent needs to spend a certain quantity of time with his or her child each day. The father who will truly invest time with his child only on Saturday morning is not emotionally committed to shared parenting.

Awareness of your role as a primary nurturer is also significant. Many fathers view their caretaking merely as "helping out"; childrearing is really the wife's job, but they are going to be nice and "pitch in." Fathers, especially, need to view their parenting role as one in which they are as deeply responsible for their child's emotional development as their wives are. A father should ask himself questions about his child and about his involvement in nurturing. Do you know your child's shoe size and the address of his or her pediatrician? Does your child like strained peaches or a particular story or song? This information is generally known by the mother because she is the parent who has traditionally been awarded the task of emotional involvement. Even mothers who have careers as demanding as their husbands' know the details surrounding their children's lives. Fathers need to become as immersed in their children as their wives traditionally have been.

Commitment on a daily basis is also an important element. You and your spouse should be equally responsible for your child's illness or for chauffeuring him or her to the baby-sitter. If an emergency develops, both parents must be equally committed to resolving it. For example, both you and your husband have scheduled appointments at nine thirty A.M. You have both forgotten about the pediatrician's appointment at nine A.M., which cannot be changed. Who cancels or rearranges his or her appointment? Who takes responsibility for the child? Your answer should not be predetermined. It should depend upon the individual circumstance. In shared parenting, problems are solved in regard to the particular nature of a given situation and not by continually attributing a certain responsibility to a specific person.

The final important emotional element involved in shared parenting is the way parents relate to each other. Even though shared parenting is never perfect, it tends to bring married people closer together than traditional parenthood does. When couples share careers and parenting equally, they are likely to have more in common and more respect for each other as people. They're likely to have a more complete understanding of the struggles of each partner in this context than in the traditional context, where the husband is often out of the house and emotionally uninvolved in childrearing. Though as parents your times alone together will not be numerous, they are apt to be more meaningful.

It is often both a surprise and a relief to parents as their child reaches his first birthday that their child is actually a year old and that they have passed through such a difficult period in both their own and their child's development. Though you may feel that you haven't learned a thing about being a parent, you most likely have learned more than you realize. At Skye's first birthday party, a girlfriend, also a relatively new mother, presented me with a box. I opened it expecting to find a pair of overalls or a toy for Skye. What I found was a blouse for myself. I looked at her in dismay. "It's my mother's tradition," she answered. "Always give the mother a present on her child's first birthday. She's the one who deserves it." Though this practice may be sexist, as it provides no gift for the father, I feel that the fundamental concept of celebrating the first year of parenthood is wonderful. Though experiencing that first year of parenting is certainly not an end in itself, it can be a milestone in our adult development. Parenting is sometimes dirty, sometimes lonely, always difficult. But through your parenting experiences, you have added a newer, fresher dimension to your life, and I hope, coupled with wisdom, you can pass the newness and freshness of this dimension onto your children.

"My Baby Is a Person."

This section does not propose to provide complete information on the topic of child development. It is a huge area of study, in which much research has been confirmed and published. What I will attempt to do here is provide some general information coupled with professional advice.

One unfortunate reaction that many parents have is to look at their newborn and expect an immediate relationship to commence. The reality is that your relationship with your child is no different from any other strong relationship; it needs to be developed over a period of time. Infants are not capable of defining relationships or developing true attachments. They are essentially selfish creatures. They want. They need. They think only of themselves.

For the first two months of life, your infant will function on one basic level—that of need and the resulting satisfaction. He does not know you are his parents. His environment—of which you are a part—swims before his yet unfocused eyes like a fog. He has not yet attributed to you any of the nurturing he receives from you. Some parents may be disturbed at this revelation, saying, "My child looked at me from his very first moment. I really felt that he knew who I was." It is true that you provide your baby with comfort and nourishment. Though the newborn has no concept of his parents, he does need their stimulation to be able to form his future image of them. Theoretically, a baby who was cared for by a machine rather than a human being would not form an attachment to the machine. Strong attachment behavior in infants is developed only through physical contact. Physical contact is important to the newborn because it is one of his few means of communication. Infants have been known to be able to tolerate certain amounts of stress better if they experience physical contact at the same time. Digestive upsets and loud noise are more easily accepted by the newborn if he is being held rather than if he is lying down.

Around the age of eight weeks, your baby will smile. As disappointing as it may be to you to know this, he is not smiling at you in particular. He is simply smiling at the human face. Almost any human face, or even a picture of the human face, will evoke a smile. Though psychologists have not yet confirmed exactly why the infant smiles at the human face, there are a few comprehensive theories available. The most widely held theory is that while the infant is being fed, he or she is often being held at the same time and as a result, can see a human face. He slowly begins to connect the pleasurable act of feeding with the presence of the human face. For a long time, the appearance of any human face will elicit a smile. The six-month-old baby often seems the most jolly of creatures because he seems to like everyone, but, in reality, he simply doesn't know who anybody is.

Around the age of seven to nine months, there is extraordinary change in a child's perceptions of other people. The parents' faces become particularly significant to him. He has come over a period of time to establish that those two faces, perhaps along with the face of a consistent baby-sitter—and of course a brother or sister—have a special relationship to him. When he discovers this relationship, he may no longer permit a new person or an infrequent visitor to attend to him. Even a grandmother, if she does not visit often, and with whom the baby may have seemed perfectly comfortable less than a month before, may provoke a howl rather than a smile at this period.

This phenomenon of preferences for specific individuals can pose difficulties for parents. One common problem is that at a child's six-month birthday often the mother returns to work and as a result needs to seek alternative care for her child. Many maternity leaves curiously are fixed at six months. This difficulty can be heightened by the appearance of another developmental milestone that tends to occur at approximately the same time—separation anxiety. Separation anxiety is your child's fear of being left by you, his parents. Separation anxiety is often viewed rather negatively by parents; it may be viewed as a sign of potential maladjustment. It is not. Separation anxiety is a normal part of child development and is indicative of healthy, not abnormal parent-child relations. This anxiety is particularly problematic for working parents whose child has been in a day-care situation or who will soon be introduced to one. Earlier in his development, a child welcomes all people into his life; now he welcomes specific people. If you have already had your child in a day-care situation, something like this may occur. One morning you take your child, when he is about seven or eight months, to the care center. You head for the door and suddenly he begins to protest violently with tears and howling. You have never seen him react this way before. You conclude that maybe someone at the care center has mistreated him or that he is ill. However, this may not be the case. He may simply be having an attack of separation anxiety.

There are several things to be aware of when dealing with separation anxiety. The first thing you must remember at this particular point in your child's development is that your child has finally realized that you are his parents, his primary care givers. He realizes that the people at the care center, no matter how loving and concerned they may be, do not have the same relationship to him that you do. Second, and perhaps more significant, is what Dr. Selma Fraiberg,[11] professor of psychoanalysis at the University of Michigan, has described as the "Case of the Vanishing Object." A child six to nine months old is an egoist in almost every sense of the word. In very simple language, if a child this age does not see a particular object in his vicinity, he concludes that that object or person does not exist. A child of this age has no concept that people and things exist outside himself. This situation may not be shattering if the child does not see his teddy bear, but if he loses sight of one of his parents he concludes not that they are simply gone for a while, but that they no longer exist. When the child's parents leave him in another's care, it can be a horrifying experience for him. To him, it appears that the ones to whom he has finally formed a strong attachment have literally disappeared.

The child who is experiencing separation anxiety will sometimes appear as if he is in mourning. He will weep incessantly or become deeply depressed or even angry.

Unfortunately, there is nothing a parent can do to relieve this terrible anxiety except consistently to return to the child. The only way a child can come to terms with separation anxiety is if the parent consistently leaves and consistently returns to the child. This constant pattern of leaving and returning will soon impress upon the child that his parents are capable both of disappearing and of reappearing. This concept, however, will not be totally ingrained until the child is almost eighteen months old. This is not to say that your child will be in constant terror of his parents leaving him for the next year. There will be times when he is only mildly upset or doesn't appear upset at all and other times when he will be severely upset by your comings and goings. The important thing is for parents to recognize their child's confusion and to be prepared to reassure him. This reassurance can be as simple as saying to your child that Mommy or Daddy is returning soon. Rather than your curtailing your excursions during this time, I recommend that you maintain your normal schedule. My reason for this is that the more opportunity your child has to experience separation anxiety, the greater opportunity he will have to cope with it and as a result to resolve it. The following are some practical points to note when dealing with separation anxiety. Never leave your child with a sitter while he is asleep. Even if you must awaken him to say good-bye, do so. Your child could awaken while you are out, and the presence of someone other than his parents could be highly disturbing. When you awaken him, simply tell him that you are going out and that you are returning soon. This action is extremely significant, since children who have awakened to a strange face have been known as a result to develop nightmares, fearing their parents will leave them during the night.

Also apparent during this time will be protestations against naps, bedtime, and parents working in a room in which the child is not present. All of these represent separation to the child. Bedtime problems are particularly evident at this time. You put your baby to bed. He begins to cry. How long should he be allowed to cry before you go in to him? How do you know if he is truly terrified? These are all questions that you as parents will have to answer for yourselves. One rule of thumb, however, is that you should not respond to every whimper. You are trying to teach your child tolerance here. If a child is never allowed to experience discomfort due to anxiety, he will never develop this tolerance. Though I know personally of many parents who will take their child to bed with them in an effort to quiet him at this stage, I do not recommend this practice. If your child awakens in a state of anxiety, sing or speak soothingly to him. Sometimes all a child needs to be comforted is to know that you are nearby, and the sound of your voice indicates your presence. Once your child is comforted, leave the room again. If your child continues to cry for longer than twenty minutes, I would normally assume that he is particularly frightened. Go into the room again at this point and plan to stay with him for a time. There are instances in which your child will be profoundly disturbed and will need your support. You can hold him and rock him to sleep or lay him on his stomach and rub his back. All these things are much better alternatives than taking your baby to bed with you. For one thing, taking your baby into bed with you is only a temporary solution to separation anxiety. It may be a helpful practice from the parents' point of view because they may be able to get some sleep, but it is not helpful to the child. He is not learning to behave independently. In addition, allowing your child to sleep with you at this time is often seen by the child as a reward for his howling. If you engage in this practice, don't be surprised if your child continues to awaken in the middle of the night. All the small child has learned in this situation is "If I cry loud enough, Mommy or Daddy will come and take me into bed with them." It must be noted that almost every parent will spend a number of sleepless nights due to the development of separation anxiety. However, this stage will pass, as do others, and will do so more quickly if you are firm and patient.

Another method of dealing with your child's anxiety is to use peek-a-boo and hiding games. These games are very simple to play. Collect a number of small toys and sit down with your child. Hide one of these toys under a pillow. At first, he may not try to find it; as far as he is concerned, the object has disappeared. Now show your child where the toy is hidden. Repeat this activity over and over again until your child begins to search for the hidden object himself. Over a period of time, your child will begin to understand that if objects can be hidden from him and yet still exist, people can too. He will become less anxious upon your leaving him in the care of another and at bedtime.

As the last quarter of your baby's first year approaches, an interesting paradox will emerge. At the same time your child is coping with the terror of your leaving him, he will actually begin to leave you. The locomotor activity of a child at nine to ten months increases significantly. Though some children are unable to walk until after they are a year old, many begin earlier. And even if they are not walking, they are experimenting. The urge to move during this stage is often so great that there is nothing you can do to keep your child still. A child motivated by this almost instinctual urge will crawl, slide, or wriggle his way across the floor undaunted by the incurred scrapes, bruises, and other threats of danger. He no longer eats or allows his diapers to be changed peacefully. He will spit, mash, and fling his food across the room, and to change his diaper often seems to require three people—one to catch him and hold down his arms, one to keep his feet from kicking you in the face, and one to do the actual changing. Sleep, though previously frightening to him, is now intolerable. He will push himself to the point of exhaustion, rubbing his eyes and angrily protesting the failings of his own body until he hopelessly falls asleep in a pile on the floor. This heightened physical activity has a corresponding effect on his personality. As his body becomes more freely mobile, his personality becomes less connected to you, his parents.

As your child takes his first step, about the time of his first birthday, he will in every sense of the word have become a person, his own person. He has awoken from the twilight of sleep of infancy to sever his umbilical cord emotionally. He is still a bit shaky and will need you for a good long time, but he has done more growing in this first year than he will do again in any other single year's period during his lifetime.

He now knows that you are his parents, but he also knows that he is somehow separate from you. As his lips form that first emphatic and sometimes terrible no, we can see indications of his potentially independent identity.

PLAYTIME

Many pediatricians now believe that the introduction of specific physical stimulation to the young child is absolutely necessary to creating secure and intimate relations between parent and child. This is not to say that your child will not develop without it but that his development may be facilitated through exercise. As I have said earlier, children are born without language, and though the human voice may have a soothing effect on the infant, his primary mode of communication with his new world is still tactile sensation. He learns about his world through the physical sensations he feels in his body.

Specific physical exercises can help your child to develop both intellectually and emotionally. As I have indicated in my previous book, *Danceplay,* motor skills tend to develop on a parallel with your child's emotional and intellectual skills. The Europeans have known and employed this principle for some time. The late Dr. Jaroslav Koch, at the Institute for the Care of Mother and Child in Czechoslovakia, conducted a program of exercise for four-week-old infants. Children who were exercised from one month on were found to develop speech earlier, have healthier appetites, sleep more peacefully, and develop coordination skills earlier than children who were not exercised. Essentially, the more physical stimulation you can provide for your baby, the greater opportunity he will have to develop the emotional and psychological effects of this stimulation.

But more important than the special developmental skills which these exercises tend to foster is the relationship that develops between parent and child as a result of these exercises. The tactile sensations that both you and your baby share will help to enhance an already close relationship. You should, of course, consult your pediatrician before beginning this program. Most infants can begin at eight weeks, but you may be advised to begin later.

To begin, have your baby lying on a soft blanket wearing nothing but his diapers. Soft music playing in the background is often conducive to a relaxing atmosphere. Never exercise your baby when he is tired or hungry. If you try during this time, he is most likely to fuss and cry. Your exercise sessions should be associated with good, comfortable feelings. If your baby begins to cry for any reason, stop exercising him and begin again later, when he is more accepting.

To exercise your baby every day would, of course, be ideal. However, if you're on a hectic schedule, it may not always be possible. I would try to set aside at least three twenty-minute sessions each week. These sessions should be shared by both parents.

The following exercises are presented with appropriate repetitions for specific age groups and with the objective of the exercise listed directly after its name.

Arm Hug

Purpose: To stretch arms and pectoral muscles laterally.

Begin with your baby lying on his back on the mat. Sit opposite him either kneeling or with your legs comfortably crossed. Clasp both of his hands with both of yours. Stretch both of his arms fully so that they are perpendicular to his body. Using your hands, bring his arms back close together and wrap them over the top of his chest.

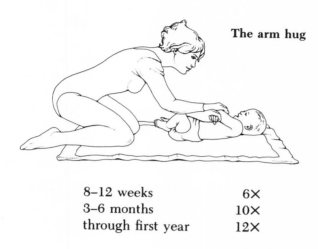

The arm hug

8–12 weeks	6×
3–6 months	10×
through first year	12×

Overhead Reach

Purpose: To stretch arms overhead.

Begin with your baby lying on his back on the mat. Sit opposite him and clasp both of his hands in both of your hands. Slowly extend both of his arms over his head, gradually straightening his elbows. Slowly lower his arms to his sides, still keeping his elbows as straight as possible.

8–12 weeks	6×
3–6 months	10×
through first year	12×

Up-and-Down Arm Stretch

Purpose: To stretch arm and pectoral muscles alternately.

Begin with your baby lying on his back on the mat. Sit opposite him and clasp both of his hands in yours. Extend his right arm over his head, gradually straightening his right elbow. Simultaneously, extend his left arm down to his side.

When both of his arms are as fully extended as possible in opposite directions, bring both of his arms, still fully extended, directly in front of his chest. Now reverse this process, extending his left arm overhead and his right arm down to his side.

8–12 weeks	6×
3–6 months	10×
through first year	12×

Heel and Toe

Purpose: To increase flexibility in the feet and ankles.

Again your baby begins lying on his back on the mat. Take his right leg by the ankle. Run your index finger over the sole of his foot, starting from the heel. As you approach the toes, you will notice them begin to curl into an arch. This is a natural reflex. Now grasp his toes with your hand. Reverse the process by gently pulling his foot back into a flexed position.

8–12 weeks	4× with each foot
3–6 months	6× with each foot
through first year	8× with each foot

Bend and Stretch

Purpose: To limber the lower back and extremities and to stretch the hamstring muscles.

Have your child lying on his back on his mat. Bend both of his knees in to his chest. Hold both of his ankles with your hands. Gently stretch his legs to their full extension, toes back. Return his legs to the beginning position.

8–12 weeks	4×
3–6 months	6×
through first year	8×

Open and Close

Purpose: To stretch the inner thigh, promote flexibility in the hip socket, and strengthen lower stomach muscles.

Your child begins lying on his mat with his knees bent into his chest. Hold his ankles with both of your hands. Gently straighten his legs into a "V" position. Now bring the insides of his legs back together. Bend his knees back in to his chest.

8–12 months	4×
3–6 months	6×
through first year	8×

Bicycle

Purpose: To increase hip rotation.

Begin with your baby lying on his back on the mat. Bend both of his knees in to his chest and hold onto his ankles with both of your hands. Slowly begin to rotate his legs as if he were riding a bicycle. When he has brought both his right and left knee in to his chest once, this is considered one repetition.

8–12 weeks	8×
3–6 months	12×
through first year	20×

Roll Back

Purpose: To stretch and lengthen lower back.

Begin with your baby lying on his back on his mat. Hold both of his ankles. Extend both of his legs so that his knees are straightened as much as possible. Lift his legs so that they are over his chest and so that his buttocks are lifted off the mat. Hold this position for a slow count of two and return to the beginning position. *Note:* Do not force this exercise. It must be done gently at first. If you sense your child is experiencing any discomfort, stop immediately.

8–12 weeks	4×
3–6 months	6×
through first year	8×

Sit-Up

Purpose: To strengthen the stomach, the arm, and the lower-back muscles.

Start seated, facing your child while he is lying on his back on the mat. Grasp both of his hands firmly and pull him to a seated position, making sure that his chin is down to his chest. Now slowly lower your child to the floor, using your arms as a support. Move your body slightly forward to encourage this downward motion. When your child has sat up and lain down once, this is considered one repetition.

Note: As you do this exercise, you will notice that your child will eventually begin to pull himself up from the lying position while holding your hands. This should be encouraged because it teaches him to use his own strength.

8–12 weeks	4×
3–6 months	6×
through first year	8×

Push-Up

Purpose: To strengthen upper body, arms, and back muscles.

Start with your baby lying on his stomach and you seated directly behind him with your legs crossed. Support his stomach, torso, and hips with both of your hands. Slowly lift your baby up off the mat, encouraging him to support his body with his hands. Hold for a slow count of two and lower him.

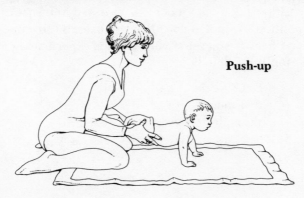

Push-up

Note: Initially your baby may find difficulty supporting himself. At eight weeks he may still have difficulty supporting his head. Be patient and give him as much physical support as he needs. Eventually he may need you only to support his hips rather than his entire torso.

8–12 weeks	4×
3–6 months	6×
through first year	8×

Perhaps due to Western society's recent glorification of the individual and his needs, the roles of family and parenthood may have been neglected. It is true that we must emotionally complete ourselves as individuals in order to be of value in any relationship. However, it is within the structure of the family that individuals are ultimately created. Society needs to support its families, if families and the individuals they produce are going to be able to contribute to society in the future. Parents need to reconsider seriously the notions they may have of themselves and of parenting in order to be more prepared to accept the responsibility they have undertaken in their parenting role, and society needs to become more involved with the needs of families. When society and the families it consists of begin to serve each other, rather than just serving their isolated interests, both will be strengthened and become more productive, and at the same time more humane.

EPILOGUE

As you finish this book, you may be comforted to know that you have everything you need to be confident and efficient during your postpartum recovery. You know what to expect biologically, emotionally, and socially. Though it was my primary intention to educate new mothers about the realities of the postpartum period, my purpose in writing this book did not end there. From a medical standpoint, I would never profess to know more than an obstetrician or a psychiatrist about the postpartum period and the complications it can produce, but many doctors and medical professionals, including childbirth educators, continue to avoid discussing this period with their clients. My hope is that their reading of this book will significantly change that situation, so that new mothers will feel secure in discussing their postpartum feelings with their physicians.

It is also my wish that women who realize that their future as mothers and as functioning individuals in society depends on society's recognition of them as equal citizens will become politically active. It will require legislation for mothers to be able both to work and to nurture efficiently. There must be more federally sponsored support systems developed and made available to every woman who wants and may need to work as well as raise as a family. The recent defeat of the Equal Rights Amendment was not accomplished by Phyllis Schlafly or other anti-feminist groups. It was accomplished by big business and a failing economy that no longer wanted the obligation to hire women. If you want this situation to change, you will need to write to your congressman or congresswoman to state your feelings on this issue. You will need to become involved with politically oriented groups, such as the League of Women Voters and the National Organization for Women. You will need to investigate political candidates, determine their views, perhaps campaign for a suitable candidate, and, above all, vote.

The term "feminism" has come to mean something more than it did fifteen or twenty years ago. Today's feminist is concerned not only with making it in a "man's world," as some of the earlier feminists were. Today's feminist wants to change some of the previously held notions of masculinity and femininity, so that both men and women will have a real choice in how to develop their lives.

Perhaps as women come closer to understanding their biological and psychological nature, and as they become aware of their potential contributions, both to their families and to society, they will be more able to help create a truly androgynous culture, where families can genuinely live, grow, and support each other.

NOTES

INTRODUCTION

1. Margaret Amelia Tauber, "Postpartum Depression, Environmental Stress and Educational Aspiration," Ph.D. Dissertation, *Dissertation Abstracts International* (Ann Arbor: The University of Michigan), 1974.

1. "WHAT ARE THE 'BABY BLUES'?" YOUR EMOTIONS

1. Margaret Amelia Tauber, op. cit.
2. R. E. Kendell, S. Wainwright, A. Hailey, B. Shannon, "The Influence of Childbirth on Psychic Morbidity," *Psychological Medicine* (London), 6, 2 (1976), 297–302.
3. Naomi Richman, "Depression in Mothers of Preschool Children," *Journal of Child Psychology and Psychiatry* (Oxford), 17, 1 (1976), 75–78.
4. R. E. Kendell, R. J. McGuire, Y. Connor, J. L. Cox, "Mood Changes in the First Three Weeks After Childbirth," *Journal of Affective Disorders*, 3, 4 (December 1981), 317–326.
5. Dennis A. Frate, Joel B. Cohen, Allison H. Rutledge, Michael Glasser, "Behavioral Reactions During the Postpartum Period: Experiences of 108 Women," *Women and Health* 4, 4 (1979.4), 355–371.
6. Harold P. Blum, "Reconstruction in a Case of Postpartum Depression," *Psychoanalytic Study of the Child*, 33 (1978), 335–362.
7. Margery Kistin Anzalone, "Postpartum Depression and Premen-

strual Tension, Life Stress, and Marital Adjustment," Ph.D. Dissertation, *Dissertation Abstracts International* (Ann Arbor: The University of Michigan), 1977.

8. Russell Meares, James Grimwade, Carl Wood, "A Possible Relationship Between Anxiety and Pregnancy and Puerperal Depression," *Journal of Psychosomatic Research* (Oxford), 20, 6 (1976.1), 605–610.

9. No author, "Postpartum 'Blues': A Special Entity?" *Medical World News*, 17, 14 (1976.2), 29.

10. J. Braverman, J. F. Roux, "Screening for the Patient at Risk for Postpartum Depression," *Obstetrics and Gynecology*, 52, 6 (December 1978), 731–736.

11. J. Hayward, B. C. Little, S. B. Carter, P. Raptopoulos, R. G. Priest, M. Sandler, "A Predictive Study of Postpartum Depression: Some Predisposing Characteristics," *British Journal of Medical Psychology*, 53, 2 (June 1980), 161–167.

12. Karen Blaker, Pfanku Lee, "Self Disclosure and Depression During the Antepartum and Postpartum Periods Among Primaparous Spouses," Ph.D. Dissertation, *Dissertation Abstracts International* (Ann Arbor: The University of Michigan), 1974.

13. Susan Kaye McCrensky-Heitler, "Postpartum Depression: A Multidimensional Study," Ph.D. Dissertation, *Dissertation Abstracts International* (Ann Arbor: The University of Michigan), 1976, p. 4.

14. Maggie Scarf, *Unfinished Business* (New York: Ballantine Books), 1980, p. 323.

15. Susan Kaye McCrensky-Heitler, op. cit.

16. Naomi Richman, op. cit.

17. Margery Kistin Anzalone, op. cit.

18. The Boston Women's Health Book Collective, *Ourselves and Our Children* (New York: Random House), 1978, p. 42.

19. B. Harris, "Maternity Blues in East African Clinic Attenders," *Archives of General Psychiatry*, 139 (August 1981), 128–133.

20. Dennis A. Frate, op. cit.

21. David J. Withersty, "Postpartum Emotional Disorders," *West Virginia Medical Journal*, 73, 7 (1977.7), 149–150.

22. S. C. Tentoni, K. A. Hish, "Culturally Induced Postpartum Depression: A Theoretical Position," *Journal of Gynecology Nursing*, 9, 4 (August 1980), 246–249.

23. E. S. Paykel, E. M. Emms, J. Fletcher, E. S. Rassaby, "Life Events and Social Support in Puerperal Depression," *British Journal of Psychiatry*, 136 (April 1980), 339–346.

24. John Jacob Seethalakshi, S. X. Charles, Abraham Verghese, "Psychiatric Disturbance During the Postpartum Period: A Perspective Study," *Indian Journal of Psychiatry*, 19, 4 (1977), 40–43

2. "WHY DO I LOOK LIKE THIS?" YOUR PHYSICAL SELF

1. Bernard J. Carroll, Meir Steiner, "The Psychobiology of Premenstrual Dysphoria: The Role of Prolactin," *Psychoneuroendocrinology* (Oxford), 3, 2 (1978.1), 171–180.
2. U. Halbreich, J. Endicott, "Possible Involvement of Endorphin Withdrawal or Imbalance in Specific Premenstrual Syndromes and Postpartum Depression," *Medical Hypotheses*, 7, 8 (August 1981), 1045–1058.

5. WORKING MOTHER OR FULL-TIME MOTHER: OPTIONS

1. Helen Harris Solomons, "Sex-Role Mediated Achievement Behaviors and Inter-Personal Dynamics of Fifth Grade Coeducational Physical Education Classes," Ph.D. Dissertation, Bryn Mawr College, 1976.
2. Jessie Bernard, *The Future of Motherhood* (Baltimore: Penguin), 1975. Mary P. Rowe, "Finding the Way to Work and Love," *Child Care Reprints*, vol. IV. *Mothers in Paid Employment*, Day Care and Child Development Council of America, Inc., 1012 14th St., N.W., Washington, D.C. 21115.
3. Marjorie Lozoff, "Changing Life Style and Role Perceptions of Men and Women Students," paper presented at Radcliffe Institute Conference, "Women: Resource for a Changing World," Cambridge, Mass., 1972.
4. Margaret Amelia Tauber, op. cit.
5. Dr. A. Regula Herzog, J. G. Bachman, L. D. Johnston, P. M. O'Malley, "Monitoring the Future: Questionnaire Responses from the Nation's High School Seniors," 1976 and 1977 (Ann Arbor: Institute for Social Research, University of Michigan), 1979.
6. Gail Sheehy, *Passages* (New York: Dutton), 1974.
7. Dr. A. Regula Herzog, op. cit.
8. Lois W. Hoffman, "The Effects of Maternal Employment on the Child: A Review of the Research," *Developmental Psychology*, 10 (1974), 204–228. F. I. Nye, L. W. Hoffman, *The Employed Mother in America* (Chicago: Rand McNally), 1963. S. R. Vogel, I. Braverman, D. Braverman, F. Clarkson, P. Rosenkrantz, "Maternal Employment and Perceptions of Sex Role Stereotypes," *Developmental Psychology*, 3 (1970), 384–391.
9. Taken from a survey conducted in 1977 by Nicholas Zill, Foun-

dation for Child Development, 345 E. 46th St., N.Y.C., N.Y. 10017.
10. Helen S. Astin, *The Woman Doctorate in America* (New York: Russell Sage), 1969.
11. Mary Dublin Keyserling, *Ourselves and Our Children* (New York: Random House), 1978.
12. Mary Dublin Keyserling, op. cit.
13. J. Bardwick, *In Transition* (New York: Holt, Rinehart and Winston), 1979. D. Lynn, *Parental and Sex Role Identification: A Theoretical Formulation* (Berkeley: McCutchan), 1969.

6. "I HAVE A FAMILY"

1. Michael Newton, "Woman, Wife, Mother: Meeting Sexual and Emotional Needs During Pregnancy," *Family Health*, 9, 10 (1977), 15–16 54.
2. Joseph H. Pleck, *Men's New Roles in the Family: Housework and Child Care* (Ann Arbor, Mich: Institute for Social Research, December 1976), pp. 38–39.
3. Taken from a conversation with Harry Finkelstein Keshel.
4. R. Rebelsky and C. Hanks, "Fathers' Verbal Interaction with Infants in the First Three Months of Life," in *Child Development and Behavior* (New York: Knopf), 1979, 145–148.
5. R. Rebelsky and C. Hanks, op. cit.
6. Dr. Jun Bay Ra's study, as reported by A. Zullo in Letty Cottin Pogrebin, *Growing Up Free*.
7. E. J. Roberts, "Family Life and Sexual Learning: A Study of the Role of Parents in the Sexual Learning of Children," Project on Human Sexual Development, Population Education, Inc. (New York), 1978, p. 43.
8. E. J. Roberts, op. cit.
9. Gail Sheehy, op. cit.
10. Gordon Hanson, "Learning Parenthood: Tending Raw Eggs," *Sacramento Bee*, January 11, 1977.
11. Dr. Selma Fraiberg, *The Magic Years* (New York: Charles Scribners' Sons), 1959.

BIBLIOGRAPHY

Bank Street Settlement, *The Pleasure of Their Company* (Radnor, Pa: Chilton Book Company), 1981.

Bach, George and Wyden, Peter, *The Intimate Enemy* (New York: Avon), 1970.

Barber, Virginia, and Skaggs, Merrill M., *The Mother Person* (New York: Schocken), 1975.

Bardwick, Judith, *Psychology of Women* (New York: Harper & Row), 1972.

Barnett, Rosalind; Baruch, Grace; and Rivers, Caryl, *Beyond Sugar and Spice* (New York: G. P. Putnam and Sons), 1979.

Bauman, Edward, *The Holistic Health Handbook* (Berkeley: And/Or Press), 1978.

Bing, Elisabeth, *Six Practical Lessons for an Easier Childbirth* (New York: Bantam Books), 1977.

Boston Women's Health Book Collective, *Our Bodies, Ourselves* (New York: Simon and Schuster), 1976.

Boston Women's Health Book Collective, *Ourselves and Our Children* (New York: Random House), 1978.

Brazelton, Dr. T. Berry, *Infants and Mothers* (New York: Dell), 1969.

Cheraskin, D. E.; *Psychodietetics* (New York: Bantam Books), 1974.

Cherry, Sheldon H., *Understanding Pregnancy and Childbirth* (Indianapolis), 1973.

Clark, Linda A., *Know Your Nutrition* (New Canaan, Conn.), 1973.

Coleman, Arthur and Libby, *Pregnancy: The Psychological Experience* (New York: Bantam Books), 1971.

Crouch, James Ensign, *Human Anatomy and Physiology* (New York: John Wiley and Sons), 1978.

Davis, Adelle, *Let's Have Healthy Children* (New York: Harcourt Brace Jovanovich), 1951.

Deutsch, Helene, *Psychology of Women* (New York: Grune & Stratton), 1945.

The Diagram Group, *Women's Body* (New York: Bantam Books), 1977.

Ditzion, Sidney, *Marriage, Morals and Sex in America* (New York: Norton), 1953.

Dodson, Dr. Fitzhugh, *How to Father* (New York: New American Library), 1974.

Eibl-Eibesfeldt, Irenaus, *Love and Hate* (New York: Holt, Rinehart & Winston), 1971.

Erikson, Erik, *Childhood and Society* (New York: Norton), 1963.

Fraiberg, Dr. Selma, *Every Child's Birthright* (New York: Basic Books), 1977.

Fraiberg, Dr. Selma, *The Magic Years* (New York: Charles Scribner's Sons), 1959.

Friday, Nancy, *My Mother, Myself* (New York: Delacorte), 1977.

Gesell, Dr. Arnold, *The First Year of Life* (New York: Harper & Row), 1940.

Gillis, Phyllis, and Lichtendorf, Susan S., *The New Pregnancy* (New York: Bantam Books), 1981.

Gordon, Dr. Thomas, *P.E.T. in Action* (New York: Bantam Books), 1976.

Green, Maureen, *Fathering* (New York: McGraw-Hill), 1980.

Heffner, Elaine, *Mothering* (New York: Doubleday), 1978.

Hotchner, Tracy, *Pregnancy and Childbirth* (New York: Avon), 1979.

Howard, Jane, *Families* (New York: Simon and Schuster), 1978.

Ikeda, Daisaku, *The Creative Family* (Japan: Nichiren Shoshu International Center), 1977.

Johnson, Virginia E., and Masters, William E., *The Pleasure Bond* (Boston: Little Brown), 1970.

Keniston, Kenneth, *All Our Children* (New York: Harcourt Brace Jovanovich), 1977.

Klein, Carole, *The Myth of the Happy Child* (New York: Harper & Row), 1975.

Lance, Kathryn, *Total Sexual Fitness for Women* (New York: Rawson Wade), 1981.

Loring, Rosalind K., and Otto, Herbert A., *New Life Options* (New York: McGraw-Hill), 1976.

Lynch-Fraser, Diane, *Danceplay* (New York: Walker), 1982.

Marshall, Dr. Edward M., *The Marshall Plan for Lifelong Weight Control* (Boston: Houghton Mifflin), 1981.

McBride, Angela Barron, *The Growth and Development of Mothers* (New York: Harper & Row), 1974.

Noble, Elizabeth, *Essential Exercises for the Childbearing Year* (Boston: Houghton and Mifflin), 1976.

O'Brien, Patricia, *Staying Together* (New York: Random House), 1977.

Pleck, Joseph H., *Men and Masculinity* (Englewood Cliffs, N.J., Prentice-Hall), 1974.

Pogrebin, Letty Cottin, *Growing Up Free: Raising Your Kids in the 80's* (New York: McGraw-Hill), 1980.

Prudden, Suzy, *Suzy Prudden's Pregnancy and Back-to-Shape Exercise Program* (New York: Workman), 1980.

Pryor, Karen, *Nursing Your Baby* (New York: Harper & Row), 1977.

Rapaport, Rhona and Robert, *Fathers, Mothers, and Society* (New York: Basic Books), 1977.

Rich, Adrienne, *Of Woman Born* (New York: Norton), 1976.

Rothman, Sheila M., *Woman's Proper Place* (New York: Basic Books), 1978.

Rozdilsky, Mary Lou, and Banet, Barbara, *What Now?* Practical guide for the first three months' postpartum period. Send $1 to the Boston Association for Childbirth Education, P. O. Box 29, Newton, Mass. 32060.

Scarf, Maggie, *Unfinished Business* (New York: Ballantine Books), 1980.

Sheehy, Gail, *Passages* (New York: Dutton), 1974.

Sheehy, Gail, *Pathfinders* (New York: Dutton), 1980.

Wheeler-Smith, Helen, *Survival Handbook for Preschool Mothers* (Chicago: Follett), 1977.

Wright, Dr. Logan, *Parent Power* (New York: Bantam Books), 1978.

Zaretsky, Eli, *Capitalism, the Family, and Personal Life* (New York: Harper & Row), 1976.

NEW MOTHERS'
RESOURCE INFORMATION

The following organizations may be helpful in assisting you with any further information you may need regarding postpartum recovery or related issues. You can also check with your Local YWCA for information regarding mother-infant programs.

BANANAS
3055½ Stattuck Avenue
Berkeley, CA 94705

Boston Women's Health Book Collective
P. O. Box 109
West Summerville, MA 02144

Center for Parenting Studies
Office of Continuing Education
Wheelock College
200 The Riverway
Boston, MA 02215

Childcare Resource Center
187 Hampshire Street
Cambridge, MA 02139

C. O. P. E.
Coping with the Overall Pregnancy-Parenting Experience
37 Clarendon Street
Boston, MA 02116

Elisabeth Bing Center for Parents
164 West 79th Street
New York, NY 10024

Family Development Program
Children's Hospital
Boston, MA 02146

International Childbirth Education Association
P. O. Box 20852
Milwaukee, WI 53220

Jewish Board of Family and Children's Services
120 West 57th Street
New York, NY 10019

La Leche League International
9616 Minneapolis Avenue
Franklin Park, IL 60131

Maternity Center
48 East 92nd Street
New York, NY 10028

Parents Center
320 West End Avenue
New York, NY 10023

Spence-Chapin Services to Families and Children
6 East 94th Street
New York, NY 10028

INDEX